WATER FASTING

HOW TO LOSE WEIGHT FAST, INCREASE MENTAL CLARITY, HEAL YOUR BODY, & ACTIVATE AUTOPHAGY WITH WATER FASTING

KATE MCCARTHY

DOWNLOAD YOUR FREE CHEAT SHEET

(<u>Don't</u> start fasting before you've consulted this cheat sheet...)

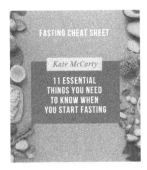

This cheat sheet includes:

- 11 things to know and to do while you are fasting.
- Why you need to know those things to start successfully.
- These things will make the process easier and more enjoyable.

The last thing I want is that the fasting process will be uncomfortable.

To receive your fasting cheat sheet, scan this QR code:

CONTENTS

INTRODUCTION

"By fasting, the body learns to obey the soul; by praying, the soul learns to command the body."

— WILLIAM SECKER (WELLMAN, 2015)

In this age of constant stress, anxiety, and increasing levels of chronic illness, many of us seek ways to repair and, hopefully, reverse the damage we have done to our bodies through living this lifestyle. While 20 years ago, the World Health Organization deemed undernutrition or starvation to be the most pressing global health issue, today we are faced with quite the opposite. Overnutrition, leading to obesity, has become the primary health concern globally, even in underdeveloped countries. Obesity is a major risk factor in many chronic diseases including cardiovascular disease, diabetes, and hypertension. The shift in this global health dynamic has led to the emergence of many fad diets and self-appointed experts who will promise you immediate, dramatic, and sustained weight loss with no scientific data or social proof to back up their claims. Sadly, these fad diets can often do more harm than good in the long term. While you may lose weight, because these new and unproven diets and eating plans are often the unscientific brainchild of nonprofessionals, you will never know what long-term damage may be done to your body. The other side of the coin is that even if these fad diets work, they will only help you lose weight, and you will not see any other overall health benefits. This is where fasting is different.

As an age-old practice, fasting has thousands of years of scientific backing and social proof behind it. Possibly one of the most well-known religious and spiritual connections to fasting is the celebration of Ramadan, which is a fasting period practiced by Muslims. Ramadan fast participants have been shown to have an improved immune response during this time, indicating the positive impact of fasting on the body. Fasting is a lifestyle that will not only help you to lose weight safely but also provide you with a huge number of other health benefits. Although fasting has its roots in ancient times, it has, more recently, gained popularity as a weight-loss and health improvement practice. This sudden surge in public interest has also led to a lot of misinformation, and it is important to clarify its roots and uses, and the actual scientific basis of how fasting works, in order for it to be properly understood and used to its greatest effect. Thankfully, fasting is the darling of the research community, as it consistently provides measurable results in clinical settings, so there is plenty of data and information to work with in making the decision as to whether fasting is right for you.

It is very likely that you already have a good idea of what fasting is, but I would like to define the concept for you from the outset for purposes of clarity. Fasting is essentially the voluntary restriction of the consumption of food to certain time periods. Fasting is not starvation, as this term implies being forced to withhold food, and it also implies that some form of damage is done to the body. Fasting is quite the opposite. When carried out correctly, fasting, as part of a lifestyle, can not only help you lose weight but also trigger and accelerate natural processes within your body that promote greater overall physical, mental, and emotional health. Our bodies are not built to be in a constantly fed state, and when we do withhold food from ourselves, our bodies react positively. Hormones are released into the bloodstream that help to maintain our glucose levels, regulate our appetite, improve our metabolic response, and even impact the nervous system.

Fasting also triggers a natural process within our body called autophagy. Autophagy is our body's way of cleaning out old, dead, and damaged cells and using that cellular material to create new, healthy cells. The process starts when we are born and occurs at a high rate in our bodies when we are young. This is why children and younger people tend to heal quicker than older people. As we age, the process of autophagy starts to naturally slow in our bodies, again resulting in the slower healing of older people from disease and injury. In 2016, Japanese cellular biologist Yoshinori Ohsumi won a Nobel Prize for his research into autophagy, which revealed an excellent method of accelerating the process no matter your age—fasting. During his study, Ohsumi found that when the body is in a fasted state, autophagy is triggered, and when it is in a fed state, it slows down (The Nobel Prize in Physiology or Medicine, 2016). This discovery has contributed to our understanding of exactly how fasting provides all of the health benefits that it does. Interestingly, the research is so compelling that pharmaceutical companies are now trying to develop a synthetic trigger for autophagy. This seems rather counterintuitive, though, as if there is a natural way to kickstart this self-healing process. There is no reason to introduce a chemical method which can only have negative side effects.

The specific focus of this book is water fasting. If you have already looked into fasting, it is perhaps important to explain how water fasting is different from other types of fasting, such as intermittent fasting. When you practice water fasting, you do not eat at all. You only consume water in order to ensure that you remain hydrated and to help your body expel the toxins and waste that the accelerated autophagy process creates. Those who practice intermittent fasting will have eating windows and fasting windows within a 24-hour period, but with water fasting, the only thing you consume is water. Water fasting is shown to have significant benefits including weight loss, the promotion of autophagy, the stabilization of blood pressure, and the improvement of the body's response to hormones like insulin and leptin.

Having explained the benefits of this protocol to you, I think it is also important for me to explain to you how I discovered water fasting and how it has been beneficial for me. I started suffering from insulin resistance in my early 20s. It affected my weight, it increased my risk of diabetes, and I thought I had no choice but to go on the medications that the doctors prescribed at such an early age. Regardless of the pharmaceutical and diet interventions, my insulin sensitivity did not improve enough to give me back the life I had previously known. This had a huge impact on me emotionally, and I felt as though my youth was being snatched away from me. Motivated to make healthier life choices, I started researching holistic and alternative practices when I turned 30. This was when I came across intermittent fasting and even more importantly–water fasting. I started incorporating both into my routine, also focusing on mindfulness, meditation, and the selection of the right foods. In time, I was able t0 lose 50 pounds. My insulin sensitivity improved so much that my doctors cleared me to stop taking medications.

Years on and in good health, I have summed up all of my research and my personal practices in two books–*Water*

Fasting and *One Meal a Day Intermittent Fasting.* I created these books with a lot of love and compassion for others, hoping that this information will help others to transform their lives and benefit from the health improvements hidden in such simple practices.

You have likely purchased this book because you have physical issues that you need to address. Such issues may include an excess weight that you need to lose, dealing with chronic illness, or simply aiming to increase your longevity and improve your cognitive functioning. My goal for you is that by the end of this book, you will have gained the knowledge and skills required to implement water fasting as a lifestyle solution to these health issues and that you will be confident enough to proceed and succeed.

Knowledge is absolutely vital in ensuring a successful water fast as it is not just the fast itself that must be specifically structured but also the prefast period and the postfast period. All three of these periods are equally important in water fasting, and that is, perhaps, one of the things that makes water fasting so different from other forms of fasting. Whereas in other forms of fasting there is definitely focus on easing out of the fast, this is emphasized greatly in water fasting. There is also significant emphasis on the prefast period and preparations for the fast in the run-up to it. If you have tried other types of fasting before, you will find that it is these preparations that make water fasting far more effective and easier to manage.

I would like *Water Fasting: How to Lose Weight Fast, Increase Mental Clarity, Heal Your Body, & Activate Autophagy With Water Fasting*, to be an all-around resource for you in your water fasting journey. It will provide you with every tool you need and answer every question you may have about water fasting. Your journey with water fasting is about to begin.

THE HISTORY OF WATER FASTING

Water fasting has been practiced since the first written record of humanity and probably even before we had the capability to produce written documents. The sudden, recent popularity of various forms of fasting may give people the mistaken impression that it is a new practice. The history of water fasting is very important to understand, though, because it reflects its synchronicity with the way our bodies have evolved and takes us back to a time when we ate in a way that was beneficial to our bodies. Water fasting was originally a very common practice which aided ancient civilizations in carrying out certain activities. Our ancient ancestors understood that while certain foods are excellent from a medicinal perspective, some of the most significant healing happens in the body when we are not eating.

FASTING THROUGHOUT THE AGES

Our ancient ancestors did not live in the constantly fed state that has become our custom in today's world. Until the first Agricultural Revolution (circa 10,000 BC), food was only available when sought out through hunting or gathering. As such, human beings would eat only when food was available, and the rest of the time they survived in a fasted state with water as hydration. It is this initial state of occasional eating that, in fact, helped us to evolve the internal energy system we use today. Our bodies started to store energy so that we could burn it when we needed to. In the Neolithic Age, man began to settle down and understand the value of farming crops and animals in one place. At this point, man began to slowly change his eating habits but still continued to eat, largely, when food was available. When the second Agricultural Revolution dawned in the 18th century, crop and livestock farming became mechanized. Even after the Agricultural Age, when food did become more readily available, civilizations still maintained a predominantly fasted state and acknowledged the usefulness of fasting in promoting good health.

Prior to the acknowledgement that fasting has an impact on our physical health, it was used predominantly for spiritual purposes as a form of soul cleansing or spiritual journey. Even at that time, though, healers and those involved in the study of medicine understood that the mind and body are connected, and what is good for one must ultimately be good for the other.

Probably one of the most famous pioneers of medicine, the ancient Greek physician, Hippocrates, included in his writings that fasting enabled the body to heal itself. He indicated that, in his opinion, to eat when one is sick is to feed your illness. This concept of not eating when we are ill is, of course, a very natural instinct within our body. Animals, too, will stop eating when they are particularly ill. Today, we take this as an indication that it's time to rush off to the doctor, but in ancient times, it was understood that this was simply an indication that the body was beginning to heal itself. Another well-known ancient Greek, the mathematician Pythagoras, who only took on disciples if they were capable of fasting for a set period, also wrote about fasting in his texts, with philosophers Plato and Aristotle also weighing in on the topic. Fasting was therefore a very popular practice in Ancient Greece and also emerged as a central practice in Ayurvedic medicine, which is still popular today and involves healing the mind, body, and soul as a unit rather than separate entities.

Greece's ancient relationship with fasting would rear its head many centuries later when Mediterranean diet guru Dr. Ancel Keys decided that it was this diet that led to the exceptional levels of health and longevity in the people of Crete. It was soon pointed out to him, though, that these same people had also practiced fasting for many generations.

Ancient warriors would use fasting during battle as they were unable to eat for long periods while they marched or fought, so they would hold off until they were camped out between battles or they had returned home in order to celebrate with a feast. It was also common for soldiers to fast before battles in order to ensure their bodies were in peak condition and that they were mentally aware. Fasting was also used as a coming of age ritual and to avoid natural catastrophes and angered idols.

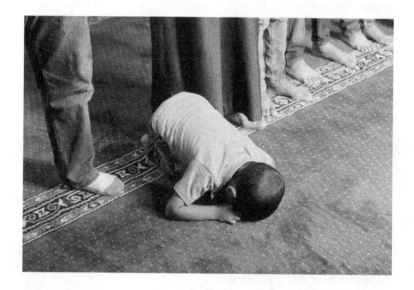

Most major world religions practice a form of fasting as part of their traditions, with the one exception being Zoroastrianism. The fast during the holy month of Ramadan, practiced by followers of Islam, lasts from sunrise to sunset each day. Water and other liquids are forbidden during the fasting period in Ramadan. Due to its extended nature, this religious fast is the most studied of all fasts and has shown that binging at the end of a fast can negate all of the good done during the fast.

Buddhists will often only eat in the morning and practice a daily fast that extends after this meal through to the next day. Buddhists also include water fasts as part of their rituals for several days or even weeks. Greek Orthodox Christians also include fasting as part of their traditions on up to 200 separate days of the year. Judaism also has several fasting days within its traditional calendar, including Yom Kippur, and Roman Catholics fast for 40 days during Lent. During the Renaissance, physicians and medical scholars wrote significantly about fasting, with one great healer, Paracelcus, referring to fasting as "the physician within." (Short History of Fasting, 2017). In reading these ancient scripts, it seems clear that even at this time they understood the great healing mechanism that is activated by fasting. Women in history seem to have linked religion or spirituality and fasting far more than men, with a practice being carried out which encouraged the refusal of food for long periods in order to prove one's purity of body and soul. A 14th century English mystic, Julian of Norwich, claimed to use fasting as a means of communication with Christ. For ancient spiritualists, it seemed that when we are able to free our minds from the binds of hunger and thoughts of food, our minds become clearer, and we are more able to focus on becoming deeply spiritually aware.

Quite separately from religion, fasting spawned itself into a method of political statement, such as that used by Mahatma Gandhi in 17 fasts he conducted in his quest to free India from colonial rule. Gandhi's longest fast lasted 21 days. The way in which Gandhi used fasts as a method of social protest is quite interesting. Another term for what he was doing is, of course, a "hunger strike," but when fasting was used by Gandhi, it was not used as a weapon to force others to give in to his demands as he "withered away" before their eyes. Mahatma Gandhi used fasting in his daily life as a means of spiritual purification, and it was not uncommon for him to fast outside of the public eye. It seems that although the public may have seen these protests as hunger strikes, it was more a way of Gandhi proving his persistence and refreshing his mind in order to continue pursuing the justice and freedom he sought for his country. Gandhi's roots as a traditional Hindi, his preference for nonviolent protests, and his vegetarianism all seem to blend well with him practicing fasting as a lifestyle rather than just a method of protest.

The Suffragettes was another famous group of social protesters who used fasting as a means of getting their point across, although for this group, it seemed far more like a hunger strike than a fast for health or spiritual reasons. The Suffragettes was a group of women in the 1900s who campaigned for the rights of women to vote. When imprisoned for their acts of protest, the women would undertake hunger strikes to force prison officials to release them. One particular Suffragette, Marion Wallace-Dunlop, began to refuse all food while imprisoned, and when a prison doctor examined her and asked her what she would eat, she replied, "My determination" (Purvis, 2009). Wallace-Dunlop was released after fasting for 91 hours as prison officials were afraid that she would die on their watch, which would result in a public uproar. If the prison officials had known anything about fasting, they would have realized that she could have continued for far longer than 91 hours as long as she had water. It is, perhaps, these hunger-strike-type fasts which have imprinted themselves on our memories as a collective and driven the narrative that choosing not to eat is somehow an act of desperation.

One of America's founding fathers, Benjamin Franklin, was a great supporter of the idea that the best medicine for most conditions is to rest and fast.

When something is known to work well, it is often skewed and manipulated to suit the needs of those with nefarious intentions, and fasting is no different. A rather dark part of the history of fasting occurred in 1912, when a self-proclaimed doctor, Linda Burfield Hazzard, formed a cult of sorts in Minnesota. The woman based her teachings and healings around the concept of fasting, but instead of using the practice to benefit people, she used it to harm them. It is believed that at least 40 patients died at the hands of Hazzard after she refused the people, who were already in very poor health, any food or water for several weeks. Thankfully, this horrendous act was a one-off occurrence, and after Hazzard's death in 1938, fasting started to move into its own as a truly beneficial health practice.

The benefits of fasting, including water fasting, were explored further in the 19th Century. The US saw a movement begin called the National Hygiene Movement, which supported therapeutic fasting for the treatment of illnesses, with the opening of a clinic by Dr. Herbert Shelton in 1928. Shelton promoted alternative medicine, including the use of fasting as a healing mechanism. He was also a vegetarian and promoter of raw eating. Shelton reported that he had helped over 40,000 patients overcome their physical ailments through fasting at his clinic (Short History of Fasting, 2017).

At the same time, in the UK, water fasts were being promoted as part of that country's own alternative medicine movement, called Nature Cure. Clinics sprung up across the United Kingdom, and some still exist in different forms today. The clinics advocated therapeutic fasting and had significant success in treating a wide variety of physical ailments. As pharmaceuticals became more widely used and people started to understand that they could take a drug for their ailments, these clinics started to wane in popularity (Short History of Fasting, 2017).

WATER FASTING IN THE PRESENT DAY

Today, different parts of the world seem to have held on to fasting more vehemently than others. Europe and the United Kingdom, specifically, have many fasting clinics that operate to this day. Tom Greenfield is a naturopath who heads up a fasting clinic in Canterbury, England. It is an offshoot of the original "Nature Cure" clinics, and Greenfield says that he still has patients that fasted at the original clinic. Greenfield admits that as medication has become more prevalent, fasting has become less popular, even in areas where it was once the go-to practice, but the patients that he has been treating for years understand and value the power of fasting and have continued its practice throughout their lives.

In Germany, therapeutic fasting is still very popular even today and is offered at various clinics across the country. German health insurance companies even work with hospitals to fund fasting promotion weeks. European fasting vacations are even popular at specialized spas and centers. The German people call fasting part of their "naturheilkunde," or natural health practice, and medical doctors in Germany are well known for prescribing fasting as complementary therapy for patients.

In the present day, we seem to have come full circle, in that we have started to acknowledge that medicating ourselves is not necessarily the best long-term solution. All chemical drugs, after all, have some form of negative side effect and can ultimately do more harm than good. It is this acknowledgement, in part, that has led us back to a focus on a natural way of doing things, including water fasting. The concepts of fasting and water fasting, in their growing popularity, have been adopted by many real experts and some pseudoexperts, who may make wild claims and promises that cannot necessarily be fulfilled. It is therefore vital to enter into water fasting armed with knowledge so that you understand what is possible and how the data backs up those claims. One of the major shifts in how we fast now compared to how we used to fast is that we are no longer able to fast as long as the ancient Greeks did, for instance. This is because of the nature of the world we live in. The many pollutants and stresses that exist in our modern world have made modern man constitutionally weaker and therefore unable to complete the extreme periods of fasting which were possible for ancient man. This doesn't mean that we can't bring ourselves into a state that is closer to where we began, though. Each time we fast, we shift our bodies further away from the unhealthy state that has become the norm for us today.

In preparing to start water fasting, it is important to understand how to do so safely and also what results you can expect. In the chapters that follow, I will provide you with actionable steps, evidence, and science-backed information regarding water fasting, and a guide to experiencing all of the available benefits. Be sure to take a slow read through the information that follows and absorb and understand the facts. In order to learn, we must think critically and actively question the information that we are given. It is insufficient to enter water fasting thinking that it's just about not eating. That very basic understanding does not help you to achieve the results you desire. In order to be successful in water fasting, you must understand precisely how the process works in your body so that you can prepare properly, fast correctly, and, most importantly, break your fast correctly.

2

WHO CAN DO A WATER FAST?

Before deciding whether to start water fasting, it is important to understand the situations and circumstances in which one should not practice water fasting. Although it is a generally safe practice, there are certain people for whom water fasting is not the best choice. In many of these situations, once the circumstances have resolved themselves, you can then proceed with water fasting. If any doubt is present as to whether water fasting is a safe option for you, always consult a doctor, and continue to gain factual information about fasting until you are 100% convinced that it is right for you. Starting a practice like fasting with doubts is not setting yourself up for success, and really, when it comes to your health, you should never do anything that you have a single doubt about. Thankfully, it is quite easy to differentiate between those who can attempt fasting safely and those who should stay away from the practice. Nothing is ever concrete, though, when we talk about the individuality of health; therefore, there is no replacement for understanding and listening to your body and giving it what it needs.

BEFORE YOU DECIDE

If you have never water fasted before, it is a good idea to visit your doctor before you start for a full health assessment. This will rule out any underlying issues that you may be experiencing which could be aggravated by water fasting. Anyone who suffers from a chronic medical condition or is on chronic medication should carefully consider whether water fasting is right for them. Also, be sure to start slowly and build your way up to longer fasting periods. It may be an interesting exercise to have a range of tests done before you start fasting. This way, you can do your own personal study of exactly how water fasting affects your cholesterol, blood sugar, blood pressure, and other body measurements.

All beginners should start with a fast that is no longer than 24 hours. Every individual is different, and the longer fasts are simply not suitable for some people. You will already gain great benefit from the initial 24-hour fast, so if a longer fast is not suitable for you, then you are not losing out too significantly on further benefits. It is important to listen to your body and be really aware of how you are feeling both during and after fasting. Successful fasting is a fine line between pushing your body into a natural state that it may not be used to and ensuring that you, as an individual, are staying within your limitations. By starting with a shorter fast and working your way up, you can find your "sweet spot" in which you are receiving the greatest benefit and also maintaining awareness of your body's limitations. It is important to recognize the difference between physical and mental limitations and to understand that both are important; however, mental or emotional limitations are easier to push through than physical limitations.

POSSIBLE RISKS

If water fasting is not done correctly, it can result in a range of physical risks presenting, and it is important to understand what these risks could be and how to avoid them. Water fasting consists of three stages—prefast, during the fast, and post fast—if any of those stages are incorrectly carried out, there are risks that can result. This is why knowledge and deep understanding of the practice and its physical impact on the body is so important before starting.

Dehydration

Dehydration is one of the most obvious risks to water fasting. Although you are supposed to take in water during your fast, it is not uncommon for people to only take in the same amount of water they would when they are not fasting, and this is where the problem comes in. About 30% of the fluid we take in daily actually comes from our food, so when we are fasting, we are already at a 30% fluid deficit from the outset. The other consideration is that most people do not drink enough water under normal circumstances, and although this may not lead to chronic dehydration when we are not fasting, it may become a problem when we do. Our ordinary eight glasses per day of water should therefore increase to at least 12 glasses per day when we are fasting to avoid dehydration.

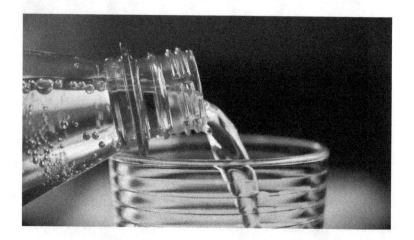

When Muslim people prepare for Ramadan (which is a dry fast), they will consume large amounts of water beforehand to ensure that they are sufficiently hydrated. They will also avoid taking part in any high-energy tasks which may result in a loss of hydration. Although Ramadan is a dry fast for religious reasons, there are those who believe that fasting for health reasons should involve no food or liquids by mouth during the fast period. Not drinking any fluid while fasting puts you at a far higher risk of doing damage to your body than water fasting or intermittent fasting and is not recommended for health or weight loss purposes. The side effects of a dry fast are also far more severe as water helps to relieve hunger, headaches, and aids the excretion of toxins through urination and sweating. During dry fasts, urination decreases significantly, which can cause kidney damage as well as urinary tract infections.

If you are water fasting and find that your urinary output has decreased significantly, increase your water intake immediately to avoid any of the added risks.

If you are a smoker and also wanting to attempt fasting, you will need to pay added attention to your water intake. Smoking cigarettes dehydrates the body, and smoking while fasting really defeats the purpose as you are continually adding toxins to a system that is trying to rid itself of toxins.

Nutrient Deficiencies

Another very common risk factor when fasting is not consuming the correct amount of nutrients. Our best source of nutrients is always food, and when we are fasting, we are not taking in those nutrients. Deficiencies can lead to a wide array of health issues. In order to avoid this, before you start fasting look for a good quality, wide-spectrum multivitamin supplement. Most of these supplements will be zero calorie but make sure you check the box or pack to ensure that they are indeed not going to interfere with your fast. Some people can feel nauseated when taking vitamin supplements on an empty stomach so be sure to drink the tablet with plenty of water to fill your stomach.

Taking supplements while fasting can also cause your blood sugar to drop significantly, which will further reduce your energy levels and increase brain fog. Some supplements may increase your insulin levels and take you out of the fat-burning process. There are also supplements that cannot work without food, and if you take them while fasting, they will pass directly through your body. The wisest option may be to discuss supplements with your doctor before starting fasting; otherwise, finding the right supplement may become a trial-and-error project and waste significant time. You will need to avoid supplements that are fat soluble as these must be taken with food. Other supplements, though, work best when taken with others, including vitamin A, D, and K. Vitamins B and C are water soluble and therefore can be taken without food. L-tyrosine is an excellent amino acid supplement which works well on a fast and helps to improve your mood and cognitive function. The following supplements are fat soluble and can only be taken with food:

- vitamins e, a, d, and k
- iodine
- magnesium
- chromium
- zinc and copper

When we are water fasting, supplements can help us to avoid nutrient deficiencies, but when we are eating normally again, it is far healthier to get our nutrients from the food we eat. If we are eating a well-balanced diet and we don't suffer from any abnormal absorption issues, then we really shouldn't need supplements. Understanding which nutrients we may be missing can be a bit of a guessing game without carrying out a battery of blood tests. Other than ensuring that your diet consists of a wide variety of fresh, whole foods, there are also some physical signs that you can look out for that are your body's way of telling you that you are experiencing a deficiency.

Iron is probably one of the most common nutrient deficiencies, and this results in chronic tiredness, a weakened immune system, general weakness in the body, and impaired brain function. There are two components to iron, one of which is found in meat and fish and the other which is found in plant-based sources. You need both, so if you are a vegetarian or vegan, then you will need to take an iron supplement. If you don't eat red meat but do eat fish, shellfish and canned sardines are excellent sources of iron. Plant-based sources of iron include beans, dark leafy vegetables, and seeds.

Iodine deficiency can result in mental deficiencies in developing children, shortness of breath, and weight gain. Good sources of iodine include fish, seaweed, eggs, and dairy.

Vitamin D deficiency can be identified by symptoms including muscle weakness, loss of bone density, and reduced efficacy of the immune system. Good dietary sources of vitamin D include egg yolks, fatty fish, and cod liver oil.

Vitamin B12 is only found in small amounts in food, so it is a vitamin for which a supplement or injection may be required. Vitamin B12 levels are also impacted by chronic medication, so anyone taking such medication should get a prescription for vitamin B12 injections on a monthly basis. Symptoms of vitamin B12 deficiency include a decline in mood and cognitive function, a lack of energy, and a weakened immune system. Vitamin B12 is found in shellfish, milk products, eggs, and meat.

Calcium deficiency is especially concerning in children and also as we age as it plays a major role in the formation and strength of bones. In older people, a lack of calcium may result in osteoporosis. Calcium is a mineral that is not well-absorbed from supplements, and we are far better off getting our intake from dietary sources. Foods that are high in calcium include dark green vegetables, dairy products, and boned fish.

Vitamin A deficiency is the world's leading cause of blindness, especially in developing countries where diets may not be well-rounded. This is uncommon in Western diet. A normal, well-rounded diet for a person in the United States, for instance, contains more than enough vitamin A to avoid deficiency. Dietary sources of vitamin A include sweet potatoes, fish liver oil, carrots (they really are good for the eyes!), and dark-green, leafy vegetables.

Magnesium deficiency can result in type 2 diabetes, metabolic syndrome, heart disease, and osteoporosis. Some of the symptoms of magnesium deficiency include muscle cramps, restless leg syndrome, fatigue, migraines, and abnormal heart rhythm. Magnesium is found in high levels in nuts, dark chocolate, whole grains, and dark-green, leafy vegetables.

Hyponatremia

This condition occurs when you lose salt and water through perspiration and only replace it with water. Although large amounts of salt are not good for us, sodium is actually an essential electrolyte in the body. It serves to maintain the balance of fluid around the cells which ensures proper muscle and nerve function. Sodium levels in the blood also directly correlate with blood pressure levels. When hyponatremia sets in, the concentration of sodium in your blood drops, and you may struggle to think clearly and develop headaches. This will not occur from normal day-to-day perspiration, but it may occur if you exercise while fasting or if you live in an extremely hot climate and spend a lot of time outdoors. If you are fasting and perspiring significantly as well, you can try to avoid hyponatremia by placing a pinch of salt on your tongue or adding it to a glass of water.

Orthostatic Hypotension

Hypotension is the medical term for low blood pressure, and it can be a very common occurrence during fasting. Orthostatic hypotension is a sudden decrease in blood pressure which occurs when you stand up or switch position quickly. The physical symptoms of hypotension include lightheadedness and dizziness. Hypotension can result from too much water intake, so it is important to find your personal requirement of water and stick to that. Hypotension during fasting is one of the reasons that it is so important to ensure that you are able to rest and not carry out any strenuous activities while fasting. If orthostatic hypotension becomes so bad that you cannot move at all without experiencing severe dizziness, it is best to end your fast. This condition can be avoided by good preparation as it is often a side effect of poor nutrition in the run-up to the fast or an excessive amount of toxins being expelled from the system.

Worsening of Diabetes Symptoms

Although fasting has been known to aid in the reduction of symptoms in many diabetes sufferers, it can also have the opposite effect in some individuals. Anyone with type 1 or type 2 diabetes should be very careful when considering water fasting and always consult their doctor before doing so.

It may be pertinent at this point to explain the difference between type 1 and type 2 diabetes so that the impact of water fasting and adjusting glucose levels can be fully understood. Diabetes mellitus, which we refer to colloquially as diabetes, is a disease of the metabolic system which results in blood sugar rising to dangerously high levels. Insulin is a hormone that helps to convert sugar into energy that is stored in our cells. When someone has diabetes, their body has one of two reactions to insulin. It either can't produce enough insulin, or it doesn't recognize insulin as what it is and can't effectively use it. When high blood sugar is left untreated or remains sustained for long periods of time even with treatment, the eyes, nerves, kidneys, and many other organs in the body can be affected and damaged.

Type 2 diabetes is probably the most common form and the form that we associate, quite rightly, with controllable causes. Type 2 occurs when your body becomes resistant to the insulin it produces, and therefore, it does not break down the sugar in your blood. The sugar levels then build up, and additional insulin must be introduced in order to reduce these levels.

Type 1 diabetes is actually an autoimmune disease and is far less controllable in terms of risk factors than type 2 diabetes. Type 1 diabetes develops when your immune system starts to see the pancreatic cells as pathogens rather than as a part of your body. These cells are responsible for producing insulin, so when the immune system continuously attacks them, they cannot do their job.

Other forms of diabetes include prediabetes, which is a consistent elevation of blood sugar but is not severe enough for a diagnosis of type 2 diabetes. In patients with prediabetes, fasting is an excellent method of treatment as weight loss is usually the first point of call for reducing the risk of developing full-blown type 2 diabetes. Another form of diabetes is called gestational diabetes and occurs, as the name suggests, only during pregnancy (Watson, 2020).

While the risk remains that water fasting may worsen the symptoms of already diagnosed type 2 diabetes, it is important to remember that water fasting can also be a powerful preventative measure in developing diabetes in the first place. If you are at high risk for developing diabetes—family history of diabetes, overweight or obese, and living a sedentary lifestyle—then a study conducted in June 2014 shows that a water fast for one day per week can help to reduce these risk factors significantly (Gunnars, 2019).

Another condition that may be affected negatively by fasting is gout. Gout is a complex form of arthritis which affects joints in sudden attacks. The treatment for gout involves maintaining low levels of uric acid. Fasting may, therefore, also worsen the symptoms of gout as water fasting leads to increased uric acid production, which is a known risk factor for attacks of gout.

Worsening of Eating Disorders

As most eating disorders develop around a psychological link between control and food, the act of voluntarily abstaining from food during a fast may trigger such disorders. Anyone who is living with an eating disorder or who has suffered from one in the past should carefully consider whether water fasting is the healthiest option for them both physically and emotionally. Eating disorders such as anorexia nervosa are extremely common in young females, and it is for this reason that fasting is not recommended in people under the age of 18, and it should be undertaken with great care in very young adults. Anyone that is already underweight or very close to underweight should never attempt fasting as it is very easy to slip under the ideal weight range simply through water weight loss. The most distinct line between an eating disorder and fasting is that an eating disorder is obsessive whereas fasting is intended to clear out the mind and body of any negative habits or obsessions. If at any time during fasting you feel that you may be developing a psychological obsession with the practice, you should stop immediately and seek medical guidance. While fasting can be a great weight loss tool, it should never be used compulsively for this reason.

WHO SHOULD NOT PRACTICE WATER FASTING

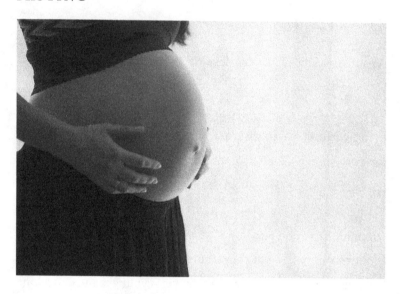

There are a few individual situations in which water fasting is not recommended. These include:

- Women who are trying to conceive or are already pregnant or breastfeeding. Women in these stages of their lives need a high level of nutrition, and the body needs to be able to focus its energy on the reproduction and gestation functions.
- Anyone under the age of 18. Children are still growing, and their bodies are developing, which necessitates a far greater need for nutrition that adults.

If you want to assist a child with better health, focus on feeding them a healthy diet and increasing their physical activity.

- Anyone who is underweight. If you suspect that you may be underweight, have this confirmed by a medical professional and undertake an eating plan that is specially developed to help you gain weight.
- Anyone with a history of eating disorders or who is currently living with an eating disorder. The restriction of food in fasting can trigger disorders that revolve around an obsession with the control of eating.
- People living with cardiovascular disorders. While fasting is good for preventing cardiovascular disorders, the sudden shifts in blood pressure and heart rate which can occur during fasting can be dangerous. Such people may also be taking chronic medication which needs to be taken with food in order to be absorbed properly.
- People living with type 1 diabetes. Those with type 2 diabetes should exercise caution when water fasting. Both of these forms of diabetes can be worsened by fasting. While significant evidence exists for its aid in relieving symptoms, the risk exists that it may have the opposite effect.
- People who regularly suffer with debilitating migraines. Headaches can be a side effect of fasting as

part of the detoxification process, and if you regularly suffer with intense migraines, this may trigger such an episode. The medication required to ease a migraine also needs to be taken with food. If you suffer from migraines and would like to try fasting, it is preferable to first seek the cause of the migraines, eliminate them as far as possible, and then try fasting.

- Anyone who has recently undergone a blood transfusion or who may have a surgery coming up that may involve a blood transfusion. This also applies to people who have recently received organ transplants. As autophagy affects the cells in your body, this may have a negative impact on someone who has received a transfusion or transplant as the immune system is impacted and may cause rejection.
- Anyone on chronic medication should consult their doctor before practicing water fasting as it is possible for certain medications to react poorly to fasting conditions in the body.
- Anyone with chronic kidney disease. When you fast, your body works very hard to remove toxins from the body. The kidneys are our main toxin-removal system, and if they are already impaired, fasting will put far too much pressure on them.

There are also circumstances which should be dealt with before water fasting is commenced. This could include periods of intense emotional stress such as grieving a death, divorce, starting a new job, or moving house. In order to be successful with water fasting, you will need to focus your mental energies on sticking to the practice, so it makes things more difficult for you if you start when you are already under severe pressure. In such an instance, wait until you have been able to move past these circumstances and then focus all of your attention on water fasting from the start.

Those who work in intense environments where focus is literally a matter of life and death, such paramedics, firefighters, police officers, and emergency room doctors, should consider starting water fasting when they are on vacation in order to avoid any loss of focus at work.

While it is nice to have family and friends who support your fasting journey, it is not absolutely necessary. You can choose whether you decide to tell people outside of your immediate family that you are fasting, but, often, doing so can just add more pressure on you. Immediate family members will likely be impacted by your fast, so while you may need to tell them that you plan on fasting, you don't need their approval. At the very least, they should just commit to not making your fast more difficult for you. Generally, you will know which people in your life are most often supportive of your choices and which are not. This is a good guideline to use in selecting who you will tell about your journey.

IS WATER FASTING SAFE?

Except for the rare few situations in which individuals should be cautious, water fasting is safe. The most important factor to consider is your individual response to the practice. Listen to your body and work within your personal health boundaries in order to achieve the best results for your situation. You know how your body reacts in certain situations, and you are the best judge of whether water fasting is the right practice for you or not. As a beginner faster, it is really not recommended that you launch into a three-day-long fast on your first try. You will still get benefits from fasting for shorter periods, so there is really no need, and it is also not advisable to push yourself too far. That said, some people would prefer to do just two longer fasts per year, for instance, rather than many shorter water fasts throughout the year. How long and how often you water fast for is going to depend completely on your personal lifestyle and what works for you. You will likely go into fasting with a preconceived idea of how you may react and what the experience will be like, and you will also likely come out the other end with a very different picture. Approach your water fast as an adventure. Adventures are exciting and interesting, but even on the most exciting of journeys, you always apply common sense and keep yourself safe—water fasting is no different. Water fasting safety should start from the minute you consider it as an option. Choose your resources wisely, consume the information you are supplied with critically and with an enquiring state of mind, and always ensure you focus on postfast behavior, including safely breaking a fast. We will delve into greater detail on the correct way to break a fast in future chapters.

3

SCIENCE-BACKED HEALTH BENEFITS OF WATER FASTING

Before we delve into guidelines for water fasting, it is imperative for me to present to you the scientific basis for the benefits that water fasting brings. This should not only give you peace of mind but also help you to understand exactly what is happening in your body when you are fasting. By understanding the mechanics of how water fasting impacts your body and how it produces the results that it does, you can also develop a realistic expectation of what you wish to achieve from water fasting. You should never attempt any health regimen or practice without fully understanding how it impacts your body. It is easy for any self-professed expert to feed you information that may seem logical. You have to live with your body for the rest of your life, though, and along with that, any damage that may be caused by following poor advice. Always ensure that you take responsibility for acquiring the knowledge you need to make wise decisions, and once you have acquired that knowledge, follow it to the tee to ensure that you are practicing fasting (or any other regimen) safely. Hype and empty promises are a dime a dozen, and anyone that would like to sell you their idea can sound convincing. Science is king, though. Empirical, fact-based data is the only way to ascertain whether a regimen is really what it purports to be. Thankfully, fasting has such research and data to back up the claims of benefits that it makes.

ACTIVATION OF AUTOPHAGY

The word autophagy literally translates to "self-eating." Thankfully, there is no cannibalism involved here, though, and the process goes on within our bodies without us even knowing it is happening. The process of autophagy involves the body breaking down and destroying old, damaged, or diseased cells and then recycling that cellular material into new, healthy cells. The process is almost constant and highly accelerated when we are young, but as we begin to age, autophagy naturally slows down. This slowing down of the autophagy process is essentially what leads to aging in humans, and the build of diseased and damaged cells contributes to diseases such as cancer, Alzheimer's disease, and other degenerative diseases. This concept is called autointoxication. Autointoxication happens when the body is negatively impacted by a toxin that it produces itself as a by-product of normal cellular function. Until relatively recently, we didn't understand how fasting regimens, including water fasting, actually caused the body to promote longevity and avoid illness, but we have now discovered the link between fasting and autophagy, which makes it clear. Autophagy, being a natural process, had for a long time been thought to be out of our control in terms of activation and acceleration. It is now clear, however, that the conditions produced when the body is in a fasted state trigger the autophagy process. As autophagy occurs in all cells in the body, this explains the overall impact of fasting on health including greater cognitive functioning as the diseased and damaged cells in the brain are consumed and replaced with healthier, younger cells. When we fast, instead of digesting food, our body can focus on digesting the toxins and waste cellular matter that are not beneficial to our health. This process of detoxification will start with the most recently acquired or developed toxins and then move on to the older toxins. Therefore, the longer you are able to fast, the more headway will be made in detoxifying your body.

Water fasting can also be very beneficial in the run up to a surgical procedure. When you activate autophagy, you will increase your rate of healing and, therefore, decrease the time it takes to heal from an operation or other procedure. The length of fast in such a case must be balanced with the point at which the procedure is set to take place. While we are ordinarily asked to fast the day before a medical procedure, this is to ensure that the anesthesia works effectively. It would not be viable or safe to end a three-day fast right before you need to go in for surgery. Preferably the fast should be completed at least a week before so that your body has time to recover from the fast slowly and correctly and that you also have time to start taking in good nutrition before you go in for your operation. Once you have been operated on and you are no longer taking heavy pain medication, where applicable, you can also embark on another fast to increase your rate of healing postoperatively. All of this should be discussed with a doctor or your proposed surgeon before the surgery.

Studies

A study conducted and published in August 2010 sought to establish the efficacy of autophagy in regenerating new and healthy brain cells. While it had been well-established in past clinical studies that autophagy cleaned up cells in many areas of the body, at this time, the medical community was uncertain about the real impact on brain cells. All clinical studies start with animal subjects as it does not require special clearance, and such studies are far less complicated than those with human participants. Basic anatomy is very similar in all mammals, though, so results gleaned from animal subjects can easily be extrapolated to human results. Researchers in this study food-restricted rodent subjects for 24 to 48 hours in order to see the impact that fasting, and as a result, autophagy, had on the subjects' brain cells. The results indicated that brain cells showed as much improvement in condition from fasting as the cells in other areas of the body (Alirezaei et al., 2010).

The link between fasting, autophagy, and possible increased longevity was explored in another study conducted in 2015. The thinking behind the link is that if we are able to replace old, damaged cells which lead to aging on a more consistent basis, then we should be able to increase the lifespan of those cells, and as a whole, the body. The connection between the build-up of damaged and diseased cells and chronic illness is also another idea behind this theory. In this study, middle-aged rodent subjects were subjected to a diet which mimics fasting in the body, and the long-term results of this were measured by comparing the postfast levels of hormones and organic compounds which are linked to longevity. In these subjects, it was found that the fasting conditions helped to extend longevity, lowered body fat levels, reduced the incidence of cancer in subjects, and improved immune system functioning (Brandhorst et al., 2015).

A third study published in 2008 investigated the link between fasting, autophagy, and a decrease in markers for chronic disease. The research determined that there is significant evidence to conclude that autophagy can help to defend against metabolic stress. It works as a housekeeper at a cellular level by cleaning out all of the unnecessary parts, reducing the build-up of cellular material in the brain which leads to degenerative brain disease, has a similar effect in degenerative muscles diseases, and can help prevent cancer (Levine & Kroemer), 2008).

AIDS IN WEIGHT LOSS

One of the main reasons that fasting has become so popular is because of its ability to aid weight loss. When done properly, weight that is lost through water fasting is not regained as is the case with many fad fasts. In order to set realistic goals for ourselves and have measured expectations, it is important to understand exactly how fasting impacts the body in order to result in weight loss.

One of the predominant ways that water fasting helps to aid in weight loss is by boosting your metabolism. When we are in a fasted state, the levels of norepinephrine in our body increase. This neurotransmitter plays a key role in boosting our metabolism.

The point that we need to get to in order to lose weight is fat burning. Fat burning for energy only happens after the glucose energy stores in our body are depleted. When we maintain a fed state, we don't give our body a chance to get to the fat stores, as it is constantly using the food that you are giving it in the form of glucose stores in order to fuel the body's processes. When you fast, though, you are giving your body the opportunity to use up the glucose stores and then move on to burning the fat stores. The rate at which fasting aids in fat burning, of course, depends on how many glucose and fat stores you have. While exercise aids the acceleration of fat burning as you are burning through energy stores more quickly than when you are in a resting state, the key to water fasting is to increase the fat burning that happens when you are in that resting state. There are domino effects to maintaining a healthy weight which go beyond self-image and appearance. Most chronic illnesses have risk factors which include obesity, including cardiovascular disease and type 2 diabetes. Doctors from the University of Oxford in the United Kingdom also explain that besides weight loss, the burning of fat for energy results in the preservation of muscle and the reduction of cholesterol levels (Gunnars, 2019).

The Academy of Nutrition and Dietetics notes that the most efficient way to lose weight and ensure it is kept off is to follow the process slowly, eat a healthy diet, and increase physical activity (Gunnars, 2019). This, of course, is sometimes easier said than done, and the struggle to lose weight becomes an ongoing, lifelong journey. One of the biggest issues with losing weight is our relationship with food. Many have developed an emotional connection to eating, and as such, we eat when we are happy, sad, or experiencing any emotion in between. It is also this emotional connection with food that leads to food addictions such as sugar, caffeine, junk food, and overeating. All of these emotional connections have a negative outcome as we begin to gain weight, become diseased, and generally feel unwell. The irony often is that the more weight we gain, the worse we feel about ourselves and the more we eat. This, of course, only leads to further weight gain and a vicious circle ensues. Water fasting can help us to reset our relationship with food. In later chapters, I will discuss the importance of prefast preparation. If you have a particularly emotional relationship with food, you will want to allocate a longer period to your prefast preparations as you are going to be using this time to start reducing your food addictions and emotional bonds to food. During your water fast, you should spend as much time as possible reflecting on how these addictions and emotional connections formed. It is not uncommon for obesity to be rooted in emotional trauma, and this is why anyone who advocates fasting understands that it is a mind and body experience. Be prepared for some issues to be raised while you are fasting that you may not have been consciously aware of, and if appropriate, seek counseling to help you move past these issues. By treating your emotional and mental health, you can significantly impact your body. This will also set you on a path to greater success in weight loss through fasting.

In order to set realistic weight loss goals, we need to consider that we did not gain the weight that we now wish to lose overnight. We will, therefore, also not lose the weight overnight. From a mental health perspective, it is important for us to set realistic goals. When we set outrageous goals for weight loss, we set ourselves up for failure and not only do we not lose any weight but we also lose hope. The best way of setting weight loss goals is by breaking them down into smaller achievable chunks that you can easily measure and setting time periods for those achievements. As you achieve the smaller goals, you can increase the magnitude of your goals and work your way up. I would recommend not setting any weight loss goal for your first round of water fasting. That initial experience is to get your body used to the practice and set yourself up for future, longer fasts. You can certainly use any weight that you may lose as a gauge for future fasts, but this should be done in the spirit of curiosity and do not be disappointed if you gain it back.

The fact that a lot of weight loss from initial fasting is related to water weight means that you are better off measuring your progress by using a tape measure to take your body measurements rather than using the scale. The scale doesn't know if it's weighing water, fat, or muscle, so it really does not give you an accurate understanding of how much fat you have lost—which is, of course, the ultimate weight loss goal.

Studies

In 2000, a study was published which sought to determine whether short-term fasting could result in the acceleration of energy burning in a resting state. The subjects of the study were exposed to a fasting state for various periods over an 84-hour period. Their levels of certain hormones, which represent fat burning, were measured on each of the days, and they showed a definite increase in the rate of fat burning in a short-term fast. It is believed, however, that if one stays without food for a long period, a week at a time for instance, fat burning levels will actually slow down (Zauner et al., 2000). The key, therefore, is to fast for just long enough to burn fat but not so long that you start to slow that acceleration or, indeed, do any damage to your body.

In 2015, researchers looked into the real impact of fasting on the body's composition. They measured body weight, cholesterol, body fat percentage, and triglyceride levels. The latter is an indicator, at a high level, for cardiovascular disease. The study looked at the impact of alternate-day fasting as well as whole-day fasting and found that in all cases, the levels of the aforementioned measurement criteria improved dramatically. Interestingly most measurement criteria did not increase significantly more on whole-day fasting than they did on alternate-day fasting (Tinsley, 2015).

REDUCES INFLAMMATION

Chronic inflammation in the body is another precursor for many chronic illnesses. Chronic inflammation can be caused by many factors including misdirected immune responses. The process of inflammation is actually the body's natural process to fight infection. It is a vital part of our immune system. It is only when that process starts to malfunction that inflammation becomes a problem. Inflammation occurs when the body sends a large number of white blood cells to the site of an injury or infection, but sometimes the body can mistake its own cells for pathogens, and this is the root cause of autoimmune diseases. When we are sick or injured, we experience acute inflammation. Depending on the illness or injury, this inflammation can present in different ways, or you may not experience any symptoms of the inflammation at all. When the body no longer exhibits a reduction response to the inflammation, and it continues on for many months or years, this is termed chronic inflammation. Chronic inflammation can also be caused by eating too much animal protein, living a generally unhealthy lifestyle, and not getting enough sleep.

Chronic inflammation results in a very high level of monocytes in the blood. Monocytes are proinflammation cells, and although they are necessary for activating normal inflammation, when they occur in excessive levels they become problematic. Researchers have discovered, though, that these cells seem to be more active when the body is in a fed state and less active when they are in a fasted state. In the latter state, in fact, they are almost in sleep mode and not producing any inflammatory effects at all. Dr. Stefan Jordan of the Icahn School of Medicine at Mount Sinai says that this discovery holds many positive implications for the reduction of many chronic disease levels (Staff, 2019). Fasting has specifically been shown to be beneficial in reducing the symptoms of multiple sclerosis, which is a condition characterized by chronic inflammation in the body.

Another indicator of chronic inflammation is increased levels of C-Reactive Protein (CRP) and cytokines, which are produced by the liver and immune system in response to inflammation in the body. After three days of regular water fasting, the levels of these indicators start to drop in the body.

Studies

In 2012, a study was undertaken to investigate the links between inflammation and several chronic diseases and by doing so, establish new possible treatments and preventative measures to limit the occurrence of such chronic illnesses. The study focused on prior research undertaken by various members of the medical research community. Research has found that patients with cancer have high levels of inflammation-related markers as well. In a study at the University of Washington, patients with tumors were monitored, and at each stage of tumor growth, inflammation markers were also measured. A direct correlation was found in the increase in inflammation markers and the growth of the tumor (Hunter, 2012). Diseases which relate to degeneration of the nervous system have also been linked to chronic inflammation. Such diseases include amyotrophic lateral sclerosis (ALS) which is relatively common and currently fatal in almost all cases.

Considering the distinct link between chronic inflammation and the occurrence of so many of these diseases, researchers started to look into how the prevention of chronic inflammation could be implemented. The use of traditional remedies and foods that have anti-inflammatory properties is an important area for researchers as these are methods that can be practiced throughout life and incorporated into the diet. A component of turmeric has been shown to provide significant anti-inflammatory properties, for instance.

Researchers also found significant evidence that fasting as well as exercise has a significant impact on reducing inflammation in the body (Hunter, 2012).

IMPROVES SENSITIVITY TO VARIOUS HORMONES

Fasting has been shown to improve sensitivity to hormones such as insulin and leptin. Insulin is produced by your pancreas and is used to regulate your blood sugar level and the nutrients that are transported by your bloodstream, and it impacts fat and protein metabolism. An intake of carbohydrates will signal your body to release additional insulin so that it can convert that food into glucose stores. In some people, the cells of the body will fail to correctly respond to the presence of insulin, and this can lead to a wide variety of issues including type 2 diabetes and other insulin resistance complications (Gunnars, 2019). Studies have shown that water fasting helps to reduce insulin resistance, thereby maintaining a steady blood sugar. The intake of any food increases insulin levels. It is possible to control insulin levels by taking in only certain types of foods that have a lower impact on insulin than others. This method, however, will prevent extremely high levels, but it will not do anything to decrease levels effectively. The key to preventing the body becoming resistant to insulin is to bring levels of insulin down to extremely low levels for periods at a time. The best way to achieve this is to fast.

Leptin is the hormone that your body releases in order to indicate to your brain that you are full and that you should stop
eating. Just like any other hormone, it is possible to become
resistant to leptin, and this is now believed to be one of the
greatest contributors to weight gain. Leptin is produced by the
fat cells in your body, and it works on the hypothalamus in the
brain to indicate that you are full and no longer require food.
This is a side-role for the hormone, though, and its main function is to regulate energy as well as the number of calories you
take in and the number of fat stores available to you. The evolu-
tion of leptin was intended to avoid us starving or overeating,
and while it has worked extremely well on the starvation end,
modern man has seemingly hacked the overeating end, and we
no longer respond to leptin's instructions in the way we should.
As leptin is produced in fat cells, it stands to reason that the
more fat cells you have, the more leptin you produce. When
your body fat increases and your leptin levels increase too, we
are supposed to eat less and burn more fat. In obese people,
though, their leptin levels have become so high that their brain
has become resistant to its signals. When your brain doesn't
pick up the leptin signals, it believes that you are starving and
will encourage you to eat more and expend less energy. By using
water fasting to increase your body's sensitivity to leptin, you
can avoid overeating and more easily control the feeling of
hunger. This, in turn, helps to avoid becoming overweight or
obese.

Studies

In a study published in 2005, researchers subjected rodent subjects to a 24-hour period of normal eating, measured their insulin and leptin levels, and then subjected them to a 48-hour fast, after which they retested their hormone levels. The subjects ranged in age from what would be considered young to what would be considered elderly in terms of rodent lifespan. Researchers found that in the initial normal feeding period, the older rats showed a lower sensitivity to insulin and leptin while the younger rats demonstrated normal levels of sensitivity. After the fasting period, all rats had the same (i.e., normal) level of sensitivity (Kmiec et al., 2005).

In another study, this time published in 2003, researchers sought to determine the impact of this hormone stabilization on brain cell degeneration. Through a mixed study which involved placing rodent subjects under fasting conditions, researchers were able to determine that the group that was fasted and showed increased sensitivity to hormones such as insulin and leptin, also showed less neural degeneration and had an overall longer lifespan than those who were allowed to eat as they pleased (Anson et al., 2003).

IMPROVES HEART HEALTH

Cardiovascular disease is one of the leading causes of death worldwide. There are several predominant risk factors to cardiovascular disease including hypertension (high blood pressure) and obesity (especially belly fat), and levels of cholesterol and triglycerides in the blood. Fasting helps to decrease the levels of these risk factors in the body and when paired with a healthy diet and improved physical activity is an excellent way to decrease the likelihood of cardiovascular diseases.

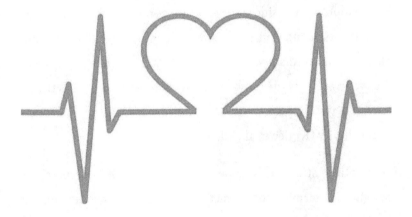

There are two types of cholesterol that exist in the body, but they are not both risk factors for heart disease. Low-density lipoprotein or LDL cholesterol is the type that we want to limit. It is known as "bad" cholesterol as it is the main source of clogged arteries. The other type of cholesterol is high-density lipoprotein or HDL. This form of cholesterol actually helps to reduce the levels of LDL in the system.

Cardiovascular disease is often diagnosed in older women, especially women who are menopausal or postmenopausal. A correlating factor to this rate of diagnosis is that belly fat is known to be far more common in women of this age range. The reason that belly fat, specifically, is so dangerous is that it is an active fat, which releases triglycerides into the blood at a far higher rate than fat in other parts of the body. Fasting is well known for its efficacy in decreasing belly fat. The presence of belly fat is one of five risk factors, which when grouped together, are referred to as metabolic syndrome. Those living with metabolic syndrome are at far higher risk of developing cardiovascular disease, diabetes, and strokes. Besides the presence of belly fat, the other four risk factors are elevated blood pressure (hypertension), high blood sugar levels, high levels of triglycerides in the blood, and low levels of good cholesterol (HDL). If you have three or more of these risk factors, you will be diagnosed with metabolic syndrome, and you will need to take urgent and consistent action to reduce the existence of these factors. Rather than waiting for too many of these risk factors to develop and a diagnosis of metabolic syndrome to emerge, it is far better to take preventative action to avoid the symptoms developing in the first place.

Free radicals can play a major role in damaging our heart as well as other parts of our body. These unstable molecules are known to cause what is called oxidative damage to parts of cells. There are foods that contain high levels of antioxidants, and these are highly beneficial, when paired with fasting, in reducing damage to the heart muscle. Examples of food that contain high levels of antioxidants include dark chocolate, pecan nuts, blueberries, artichokes, strawberries, raspberries, kale, and goji berries.

Hypertension or high blood pressure is one of the leading contributing factors to cardiovascular disease.

Studies

In a study conducted with a group of 68 people, all of whom suffered with high blood pressure issues, the participants were subjected to a fast for almost 14 days while under constant medical supervision. At the end of the period, 82% of the participants had reduced their blood pressure to normal levels (Gunnars, 2019)

In one study, 30 participants who presented as healthy adults were subjected to a water fast for just 24 hours. Their levels of cholesterol and triglycerides were measured before and after the 24-hour water fast, and it was found that their postfast levels were significantly reduced (Raman, 2019).

In another study, 174 participants suffering from hypertension were subjected to water fasting for 10 days, again under medical supervision. At the end of the 10-day period, 90% of the participants had seen a drop in blood pressure to readings that are considered normal (Raman, 2019).

In 2007, a study was undertaken to determine the impact of fasting on blood pressure, cholesterol, and triglycerides in the blood. Researchers used a group of 110 patients with a mix of male and female patients, all of whom presented with obesity. The patients were hospitalized for the duration of the study and were subjected to fasting conditions. Their blood pressure, cholesterol, and triglyceride levels were monitored before, during, and after the fasting was complete. At the end of the three-week period, all subjects had lost up to 40 pounds each. Their blood pressure levels had dropped to a normal reading, and their cholesterol and triglyceride levels had all decreased significantly (Beleslin et al., 2007).

PREVENTION OF DEGENERATIVE DISEASES AND COGNITIVE DECLINE

The degenerative diseases which are often linked with age such as Alzheimer's Disease are often seen as almost an inevitable part of ageing. The truth, though, is that scientific research is discovering that it is entirely possible to take preventative measures throughout our lives in order to significantly reduce the possibility that we will present with these diseases in old age. The basis of this idea is the link between the build-up of damaged and diseased cells and degenerative disease as well as general cognitive decline. The reason this build-up happens is because of the naturally slowing rate of autophagy in the body as we age. The body is less capable of removing damaged and diseased cells from all areas of the body, including the brain, and this build-up plays a role in cognitive decline and disease.

As we know, fasting is a trigger for autophagy, and this is the reason that we now see fasting as a preventative measure in avoiding cognitive decline and disease. Although this benefit may only seem apparent in later years, it is widely recognized that fasting boosts cognitive functioning in people of all ages. It is particularly beneficial for women who are experiencing brain fogging due to hormonal changes such as after pregnancy and during menopause. Women who have given birth should always wait until they have stopped breastfeeding to start fasting.

The link between our cognitive functioning and food, or the absence thereof, becomes clear if we consider what our own cognitive functioning is like around food. When you eat a large meal, you start to feel tired and incapable of performing cognitively. Often, you will need to go and have a nap in order to feel better. This is because, when you overload your stomach with food, your body automatically shifts the majority of blood flow to the digestive system in order to aid digestion. As a result, your brain is left to function on minimal blood flow, which is generally just enough to keep messages flowing to your muscles and organs. You feel the need to sit still or lie down as a result of your body wanting to direct that blood flow elsewhere. By the same token, when you don't eat, you feel mentally sharper. You may become hyperaware and find it easier to focus. This is physical proof of our brain's relationship with food.

There is a wide range of diseases which are considered to be degenerative in nature. These include:

- Alzheimer's disease
- Cancers

- Amyotrophic lateral sclerosis (ALs), also known as Lou Gehrig's disease
- Charcot-Marie-Tooth (CMT) disease
- Cystic fibrosis
- Chronic traumatic encephalopathy
- Huntington's disease
- Frontotemporal dementia
- Macular degeneration
- Parkinson's disease
- Rheumatoid arthritis
- Motor neuron disease

A disease is considered degenerative if it results from a consistent degradation of cells in the body which impact the functioning of organs or tissue. Once a degenerative disease has manifested, it can, in most cases be treated in terms of the symptoms, but degeneration will continue and there are no cures for most of these diseases. Many will have fatal results. The need for preventative measures cannot be overstated, especially if you already have risk factors for these diseases. If you are genetically predisposed or your lifestyle habits make you more likely to develop one of these degenerative diseases, it is imperative that you act beforehand and give your body the best chances of fighting off such a disease.

Studies

In 2013, a study was published which delved into the impact of fasting on cognitive development and functioning. The study was conducted over 11 months and started with young rodent subjects in order to track their brain development and cognitive functioning levels when exposed to different diets. One group was submitted to a constant intermittent fasting diet while the other was fed on a high fat diet. The subjects' cognitive abilities were tested throughout the study period, and by the end of the study, it was determined that the group that had been subjected to the fasting diet had far better cognitive and problem-solving abilities than the group that had been subject to the high-fat diet. There was no difference in the way the brain developed in terms of structure, but there was significant difference in the way the rodents were able to think and solve problems (Li et al., 2013).

Another study conducted in 2000 sought to determine whether the generation of new brain cells could be impacted by restricting the intake of food—in other words, fasting. Adult rodent subjects were put into a fasted state for intermittent periods of time during the study. The levels of new brain cell generation as well as the release of Brain Derived Neurotrophic Factor (BDNF) were measured. BDNF is a hormone that when present in higher levels is known to increase the rate of neural cell generation. All subjects showed increased levels of all tested criteria after fasting (Lee et al., 2000).

INCREASED SECRETION OF HUMAN GROWTH HORMONE

Human Growth Hormone (HGH) is a hormone produced by your pituitary gland that plays a key role in the body. It is involved in growth, weight loss, metabolism, and muscle strength. Levels of HGH decrease in the body as we age, and this is one of the reasons that older people find it more difficult to lose weight and experience muscle wastage and loss of strength. Your diet and lifestyle can impact the levels of HGH in your body at any age.

Research has shown that water fasting could help to increase HGH levels in the body, regardless of age. The ability of water fasting to help maintain steady blood sugar and insulin levels also helps to increase levels of the hormone, as consistently peaked insulin levels have been shown to reduce HGH in the blood.

HGH is also increased further by losing body fat, and there is a direct correlation between the amount of belly fat in the body and the levels of HGH. The more belly fat that a person has, the lower their levels of HGH. Arginine is a supplement that can be taken while water fasting that helps to increase HGH levels as well. If you are specifically looking to increase your HGH levels while water fasting, use your preparation time to cut out all of your sugar intake. When sugar levels are high, so is insulin and as a result HGH is suppressed. The time at which you eat when you have broken your fast also makes a difference in your HGH levels. Eating too close to bedtime is not only bad for your digestive system, but it reduces your HGH levels.

Studies

In 2012, researchers were able to determine that during a 24-hour fast, levels of HGH increased in study participants. Another study also showed that levels of HGH increased by five times the nonfasted level, in participants who were subjected to a 24 to 48-hour fast (Salgin, 2012).

In one study conducted over one week of fasting, researchers found that within three days of fasting, participants' HGH levels had increased by 300%. After a full week of fasting, these levels had increased by 1,250%. Other studies indicated a tripling of HGH levels after just two days of fasting (Salgin, 2012).

APPLIED BENEFITS

The benefits of water fasting and autophagy can be applied in several areas to improve health. Researchers are now looking at using fasting as a complementary treatment for cancer patients who are on chemotherapy as it helps to improve the removal of dead and diseased cells and replace them with healthy cells that are more likely to fight the disease. Fasting may also make chemotherapy more effective in the body while reducing the side effects of the treatment. A study conducted on the growth of tumor cells showed that cyclical fasting was as effective as chemotherapy in retarding the growth of tumor cells. Medical advice should always be sought before commencing fasting as a complementary treatment while taking chemotherapy.

Water fasting can also be beneficial in many autoimmune diseases as it helps to reboot the immune system and may reduce the symptoms of several autoimmune diseases such as inflammation. When you incur an injury or suffer from a disease, your body sends white blood cells to the site in question to aid in healing. White blood cells, just like other cells of the body, have a limited lifespan, and as they age, they become less effective. Stem cells are those that give rise to new white blood cells, and it has been shown that water fasting activates stem cells to produce new white blood cells and rejuvenate the immune system. A significant figure in the fasting research community, Dr. Valter Longo, conducted a study with a research team from the University of Southern California to investigate the true impact of fasting on the immune system. The team found that water fasting of between two and four days in length can renew many of the cells in the immune system and effectively reboot it. Dr. Longo explains that when you do not take calories in, your body saves energy by recycling many of the cells of the immune system that are not required as well as those that may be damaged or ineffective. Longo went on to demonstrate that in people whose immune systems are already significantly damaged, such as those on chemotherapy, this process can effectively rebuild an entire immune system (Gunnars, 2019).

The process of autophagy, which replaces dead and diseased cells with new cells, will also have the applied benefit of increasing overall longevity. While this theory has only been tested and proven in animal subjects, the science behind the theory certainly indicates that the same would be applicable to humans. The fact that water fasting and autophagy definitely reduce our risk of developing several chronic diseases also contributes to the idea that lifespan would be increased by this practice.

From the perspective of appearance, wrinkling and sagging of skin occur as we age predominantly because our body produces far less collagen than it did when we were younger. Collagen is a protein in the blood that helps to provide structure to the skin and aids in the clotting of blood. Fasting has been shown to promote healthier levels of collagen in the skin, thereby improving skin structure and appearance.

Overall, fasting helps to improve our relationship with food. If you really sit and consider how much time you spend every day thinking and talking about, and preparing food, you will likely be amazed at how much of your time it takes up. When we structure our eating by water fasting, we free up our minds to focus on other areas of our lives. The modern way of eating, which basically involves being in a constantly fed state, has damaged our relationship with food. Rather than seeing food as something that nourishes our body, we have started to see it as something that we need to have constantly available to us. In some cases, this can actually lead to emotional disorders developing around food where it is used as an emotional crutch. This constantly fed state has also impacted our understanding of hunger. Most human beings today do not understand what true hunger is or what it feels like. We mistake boredom, emotional disturbance, and even thirst for hunger. By implementing water fasting as a lifestyle, we can reset our brain's understanding and response to true hunger and help our bodies to reach a more natural state in this regard.

Water fasting, in particular, has additional applied benefits to ordinary intermittent or other forms of fasting. Water, of course, is an extremely important substance to the human body. When we drink water, it is not absorbed in the same way that food is. While food is digested, water is absorbed directly into our system. This rate of absorption is far higher when our stomach is empty, though. Drinking water improves hydration levels, energy level, and physical performance. It also supports the growth of hair and the composition of skin. Water is absolutely necessary to ensure that functions in the body, including brain function, continue correctly. This is one of the reasons that when you start to become dehydrated, you also develop a brain fog. Severe dehydration can even lead to hallucinations as your brain functions start to completely shut down. Several forms of headaches and migraines can actually be caused by not having sufficient hydration levels, which is why doctors recommend drinking a large glass of water before taking any pain medication for a headache. After waiting about half an hour, you will be able to see whether there is any easing of pain, and if so, you will know that your headache was actually caused by dehydration. When we fast and increase the autophagy process, we produce more waste material that needs to be removed. Our kidneys are the predominant organ involved in flushing toxins from our bodies. In order for our kidneys to work efficiently, they need water. Sweating is another way that our body gets rid of toxins, and water is also required for this process. The more we sweat, the more we need to replace that lost fluid by drinking more water.

In comparison to other plans which simply require a restriction of calories, fasting has been found to be far more effective at reducing weight while, importantly, preserving muscle tissue. Water fasting is also a far safer way to induce ketosis (fat burning) in your body. It avoids a state called metabolic acidosis which can be common in low-carb, high-fat diets. Metabolic acidosis occurs when ketones build up in the body due to ketosis being too quickly achieved for too long a period. The kidneys struggle to remove these ketones and their resultant acid from the body and, as a result, the body slowly begins to be poisoned.

Another resultant benefit of fasting is that your body intuitively knows where to send blood, and when you are fasting, your digestive system, which usually uses the largest supply of blood, no longer needs it. As a result, increased blood flow is sent to your lungs and skin, both of which are excellent organs of detoxification.

The emotional and mental health benefits of fasting are significant and proven. When the detoxification process starts to occur and fat is burned for energy, we experience a state in our body which is similar to exercise. Endorphins or "feel good" hormones are released at this stage, and this results in an intense feeling of well-being and happiness. A reduced rate of endorphin production is one of the risk factors for mental health diseases like depression and anxiety. Mental health disorders like these affect at least 25% of the global population. The release of additional BDNF as well as the decreased levels of inflammation in the body have both been shown to aid in reducing the severity of depression. Many pharmaceutical antidepressants work to increase the level of BDNF in the body, and while it is not intended to replace antidepressants at all, fasting may definitely help in making their work easier. Another interesting link can be made between the impact that fasting has on the helpful bacteria in our gut and our mental health and brain activity. The bacteria that live in our gut are called microbiota, and they play a surprising role in our body. Microbiota are not just useful in aiding digestion; they also play a role in sending signals to the immune system to maintain its proper functioning and in turn influence levels of inflammation, which plays a role in depression. A direct link between the gut and the brain has been established, and imbalances in one have been shown to directly impact the other. The benefit of fasting in restoring gut health is, therefore, another way in which it plays a role in mental health (Rose, n.d.). Fasting should never replace psychotherapy or pharmaceutical aids in people suffering from severe depression or anxiety, but it can certainly play a role in aiding the reduction of symptoms.

4

GETTING STARTED WITH WATER FASTING

As with any new journey which aligns with specific goals, planning is imperative to ensure that you can reach your goal safely. Water fasting is no different. In order to get the best results possible out of water fasting and to practice it safely, it is important to understand the prefasting practices which should be followed. By following the preparation steps which I will lay out in this chapter, you will radically improve your chances of success.

WHAT TO CONSIDER BEFORE WATER FASTING

Setting a time period for your first water fast should be determined by your experience in fasting. If you have never fasted before, it is better to start with a shorter period and work your way up. A 24-hour period should be sufficient to start, but if even that sounds a bit too much to begin with, feel free to start on a shorter period and slowly increase. The reasons for starting small and working up are several. You will experience some side effects as your body starts to adjust to no longer being constantly fed, and by building up your fasting period, you give yourself an opportunity to slowly work through those side effects rather than experiencing them all at once. Many people who fail at water fasting try to go for too long a period on their first occasion, and when they suddenly experience many side effects at once, on top of dealing with hunger, the experience becomes overwhelming and they quit. If you had no experience with running, you wouldn't go out for a 20-mile jog on your first day, would you? You would start with a walk around the block and then a run, and then you would build up your distance bit-by-bit. The same concept applies to fasting. Water fasting may not be exercise in the true sense of the word, but just as exercise puts a form of stress on your body (good stress in this context), so does fasting. That is why it is vital to get your body used to this new way of being slowly and gradually.

If you are currently in a constantly fed state, you put yourself at risk for nutritional deficiencies by suddenly reducing your food intake. This is another reason that your run-up to the water fast is so important. A good way to start is with one 24-hour water fast per week. After a few weeks of successful 24-hour water fasts, you can start to build yourself up to a 48-hour fast. Those who are obese or suffer from chronic inflammation can try and build up their fasts to longer than three days, keeping in mind that your body needs to get used to consuming only water, and many people may not cope well with extended periods of water fasting.

Educating yourself about water fasting is one of the most important parts of preparation. By reading this book, you are doing exactly that. As I have mentioned in other parts of this book, if you are living with a chronic condition or take prescription medicine, it is important to consult a doctor before starting water fasting, just to ensure that you understand how a fasted state might interact with your medication or condition.

PICK YOUR MOMENT

Water fasting is not something that can be done on the spur of the moment due to its intensity. You will need to choose a time when you are not experiencing any major stress or changes in your life. It is also preferable to be able to spend most of your time in a rested state while you are fasting and not undertake any strenuous activities. Your body is going to be in a major period of healing and repair, and it needs to be able to focus the bulk of its energy on carrying out those internal activities.

If you are feeling physically or emotionally unwell, do not start your water fasting at that time. Use your fasting time to enrich your mind and soul. Spend time reading, enjoying the company of pets, and sleeping as much as you can. Your body heals really when you are asleep as it doesn't need to expend energy on thinking or moving muscles. A good time to start water fasting could be over a weekend or when you are on vacation and spending time at home.

If you want to do an extended fast and aren't able to take time off work, then you can attempt the fast with your normal routine, but this is not recommended for first-time fasts. You will not know how your body is going to react until you start fasting, so it really is better if you allow yourself time to adjust in a safe space.

PREPARE YOUR BODY

The changes that your body is going to undergo when you are water fasting are quite dramatic and, in order to get the most out of the fast, it is important to ensure that your body is prepared for the water fast beforehand. Think about it as preparing yourself for battle. In the days before your water fast, you will need to be really selective and purposeful about what you put into your body. Your body cannot make the changes it needs to if you have fed it junk beforehand. Also consider that one of the main processes you want to accelerate is the burning of fat, and in order to get to that stage, you need to burn through your glucose stores first. If you eat a lot of processed and refined carbohydrates in the days before your fast, your body will have a lot more glucose stores to work through before you get to the fat-burning stage. This clean and healthy eating preparation period should last at least one week before your fast (two weeks if you can manage it). An easy way to do this is simply by reducing the number of unhealthy snacks or treats you allow yourself per day and start to reduce the portion size you are consuming when you eat. You want to give your digestive system the best chance possible to perform well during a fast, so it is important to avoid difficult to digest foods such as animal proteins and dairy products in the preparation period before your water fast. Plenty of fruit and vegetables are vital for their nutrients and fiber content. Organic produce is always best as you are ensured that you are not taking in chemicals or the like, but if you are unable to get organic, as long as the produce is fresh, that is completely fine. Increase the amount of antioxidant-rich foods you take in during your preparation period to ensure that the destruction of free radicals is optimized during your fast.

During this preparation period, get into the habit of increasing your hydration and relying on water as a substitute for food. This will make it much easier for you when you start water fasting as your brain will already be accustomed to seeing water as satisfying. This is also a good time to prepare the quality of water that you plan to drink during your fast. Depending on the area you live in, you might have access to decent quality tap water. Even if it is drinkable, though, tap water rarely contains the same amount of minerals that bottled water does. Bottled water can get expensive, though, so you should consider investing in a high-quality reverse osmosis filter system for your home so that you can convert tap water to high quality water within the comfort of your own home at no cost to you. Salt as electrolytes is also an important consideration, and the quality of salt you consume also makes a huge difference. You can use this preparation time to find the best quality salt that you can afford. The best salts are ideally sea salts, and you can add some to your drinking water to get in those much-needed electrolytes.

One of the best ways to get in a lot of fresh produce and ease up on your digestive system is by drinking vegetable and fruit smoothies in the run up to your fast. Smoothies are also a great way to take in natural anti-inflammatories like turmeric. It may be a good idea to ease your body into water fasting by drinking smoothies only for a day or so before you commence your fast.

Also during this period, try to reduce anything that you may take in that could result in toxins in your body. This includes alcohol, cigarettes, refined sugary drinks, and any over-the-counter medication that you may take regularly. The intensity of the side effects you experience during water fasting will be in direct correlation to the amount of toxins you are putting into your body just before the water fast. If you live a high-toxin life-style such as smoking, drinking an excessive amount of alcohol, eating poorly, and not exercising, you can expect to experience a significant number of high-intensity side effects if you go straight from that lifestyle into water fasting. This is why I highly recommend taking a week or two before you start your first water fast to gradually change your lifestyle and allow your body to start moving those toxins out.

Some experts recommend starting with intermittent fasting in the days before your extended water fast starts as this can start to prepare your body to enter ketosis more quickly. Intermittent fasting is when you have a fasting window and an eating window within the same 24-hour period.

GET MOVING MODERATELY

Moderate exercise is a very beneficial part of your preparation for a water fast. Select activities that you look forward to doing so that you are maintaining good emotional stability. Yoga and meditation are both great for your prefast preparation as they exercise both the mind and the body and help you get into a centered and mindful place, which will be vital for a successful fast. A daily walk in the park (with a dog if you have one) has a calming effect which helps to reduce stress levels. It is important to avoid really strenuous exercise in the period before your water fast, and also while you are fasting. Ensure that you get lots of sleep and rest in this period as well.

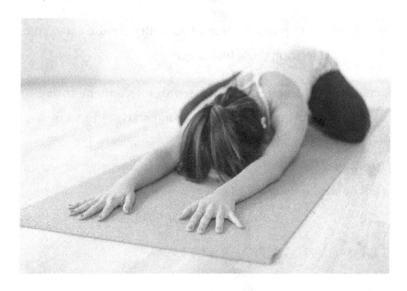

Yoga is an exercise that fits in really well with the fasting lifestyle. Its focus on mindfulness, breath exercise, and meditation
is beneficial in keeping the mind focused during fasting. You
don't need to go to a yoga class to enjoy yoga. There are many
online classes as well as DVDs focused on teaching yoga to
beginners. Meditation is a mind exercise that is really helpful in
staying focused on your goals. While you may picture a monk
sitting cross-legged in a temple when you think about meditation, it is really much simpler than that. The point of meditation
is to clear your mind and be present in the moment. To do this
you will need a quiet area. The idea behind meditation is that
you don't need to push things out of your mind. As you sit and
focus on your breathing, ideas, thoughts, and emotions will
inevitably pop into your head. When they do, don't become
frustrated with yourself; simply acknowledge the thought or

emotion without judgment and allow it to move on. This concept of mindfulness is very helpful in reducing any anxiety you might feel about the water fasting process. It is almost impossible to feel any anxiety if you are in the present moment. Anxiety is about past and future events, not current events, so if you are focused only on what is happening right now, anxiety is not a concern. When you are fasting, mindfulness is a great tool to keep you grounded and centered. If you don't already practice mindfulness or meditation, try to include this in your preparation period so that you can be adept at it during your water fast.

Stretching is another great exercise during your fast. It is a low-impact exercise but really helps to improve flexibility in your muscles and get your blood flowing. Stretching will be especially beneficial if you are used to high-impact exercises under normal circumstances and you are missing that while you are fasting. By stretching twice daily, you will keep your muscles supple and reduce stiffness. Stretching is particularly good for those over 40 who may start to experience the aches and pains associated with age. Back pain is one of the most common complaints in people of that age group, and stretching can help to improve the strength of core muscles and encourages better posture, which is often the root cause of back pain. Stretching exercises are a surprisingly good stress reliever and, as with yoga, as you begin to focus on the movement of your body and your breathing, it's easier to move the stresses of the moment out of your mind. If you are struggling with headaches during your fasting, stretching may help to relieve them as well. If you are new to stretching, there is a proper form that you need to follow in order to avoid injury. There are several online resources and books that will teach you the correct way to stretch and give you an idea of what sort of stretching you should be doing. Stretching is rather more involved than the stretch you do when you get out of bed in the morning so be sure to do your homework and some research before starting.

PREPARE YOURSELF MENTALLY

It is often the unexpected side effects of a water fast that cause people to fail. If you have an unrealistic expectation of what fasting will be like, and then you are met with a very different reality, this may be the cause of failure. Hunger is probably the biggest obstacle for most people when they fast for the first time as the body and mind have not yet adjusted to the true nature of hunger. Keep in mind that your body is used to constantly being fed, so the sudden absence of food could well produce signals in your brain that are similar to the fight-or-flight reaction. Your brain tells your body that something must be very wrong because you haven't fed it in several hours. It will likely increase the amount of ghrelin (hunger hormone) that it produces so that you can't miss the message that you "need" to eat now. Work your way through this possibility before you start fasting and get yourself to a point of acceptance. It is important for us to accept and understand that the messages our brain will send us during this initial fast period are essentially false. Try to get to the point where you see past these mixed messages and continually tell yourself that you are simply in transition and that, on the other side of your fast, your brain will start to return to its natural state of true comprehension of the hunger signal. If you have prepared your body with healthy and clean foods in the run-up to your fast, then you consciously know that you have everything you need to get through your water fast.

It is not uncommon to feel lightheaded, dizzy, and sometimes nauseated during your first fast. These are signs that your body is adjusting to a new way of being, and, as you know, a more natural state of being. This is why it is important to ensure that you don't have a lot going on when you plan to fast so that you can rest when you need to deal with these symptoms. Due to the change in food intake, you can also expect your bowel movements to change. There is no need to be alarmed if this happens as it should return to normal fairly quickly. If you are constipated, there is a possibility that you are not drinking enough water, and you should consider increasing your water intake. While we are on the topic of toilet habits, it is possible to drink too much water, and the color of your urine is a good indicator as to whether you are drinking too much or not enough water. Very dark, pungent-smelling urine is an indicator that you are not drinking enough water while completely clear urine means you are drinking too much water. Urine should not have an intense odor, and it should be light in color but tinged yellow.

With regards to weight loss, it is important to have realistic expectations upfront. You are not going to get to your goal weight after one round of fasting. When you fast, your body begins a process of burning through glucose, then fat, and it will become more efficient at doing this, the more you expose it to a fasted state. It is also important to keep in mind that while you may lose pounds on the scale, that does not necessarily equate to body fat. The scale cannot determine what type of weight you are losing, and it is very likely that on your first fast, you will predominantly be losing water weight. Temper your weight loss goals with the acknowledgement that you have started somewhere. Even if you do a 24-hour fast and don't lose a single ounce on the scale, you have initiated processes in your body that are setting you on the right path. Water fasting is not a once-off deal. You need to practice it as a lifestyle in order to get the best benefits from it and that includes weight loss. The way you eat in the run-up to your water fast is also any important part of your weight loss, and if you keep up a healthy diet and clean eating, you will undoubtedly start to shed the extra pounds quickly. Physical activity outside of your fast is also important to encourage weight loss.

Some other side effects that you may experience during fasting include increased body odor as sweating increases to remove toxins from your body, and headaches.

Part of preparing yourself mentally is ensuring that you know why you are doing this. Having a deep visualization of what you want to attain from your fast will help you to keep going when things get rough. For every difficult symptom that you may encounter, there is probably no better adage to keep in mind than "this too shall pass." It really will, and you will likely be surprised at how quickly the negative side effects of fasting do pass. If you are able to keep your goal in mind and continually remind yourself why you decided to fast in the first place, you will be far more likely to succeed. Another great way to prepare yourself mentally is to plan something that you enjoy (not food related obviously) right in the middle of your planned fasting period. A spa day, for instance, is a good example as you will be relaxing and pampering yourself without involving any food.

One of the most important things you will need to do while water fasting is to trust your body. While we like to think that our body and mind are separate, they are not. Our mind does not control our body or vice versa—they work in unison. Your body knows what it needs. This is what we need to learn to trust. Although we may have gotten ourselves to the point as a society where we ignore our body's signals or find ways to mask them so that we don't have to listen, our body continues to communicate its needs. Water fasting is about using your internal intuition to know when to stop and also using your success in fasting to reconnect with your body and begin to trust its judgment again. Perhaps the best explanation of trusting your body is the feeling you get in your gut when you know something is not right. We have all had it, and many of us have ignored it to our peril. Although we ignore the signals that our body gives us, it knows and understands far more than our conscious mind is able to comprehend—we just need to quiet down and listen.

You know yourself better than anyone else, so a big part of successfully preparing yourself for this water fast will be figuring out where you have gone wrong in the past and correcting those mistakes now. Some people cannot be around temptation at all, and if you are one of those people, then in order to succeed, you need to ensure that you keep yourself away from anything or anyone that is going to tempt you to break your fast. Other people may have greater self-discipline in staying away from temptation, but their weakness may be over-thinking and creating anxiety for no reason. In your mental preparation phase, ask yourself what you usually do to self-sabotage and what you can do this time to avoid doing so. If you haven't tried any other health regimens before, then you may not have any information about how you react in such situations. If that is the case, then your water fast will be a self-discovery journey as well. Take special note about your emotional reaction to the different parts of the fast, and if you happen to find it difficult to reach your goal the first time round, dig deep to understand why and how you can change that in the future.

Although it is important to push yourself as much as possible and not fall at the first hurdle, you also don't want to do any damage to yourself. As with any other dietary lifestyle or practice, water fasting is not for everyone. If you start to feel very uncomfortable or experience changes in your heart rate or breathing, discontinue your fast immediately and undertake medical advice.

A journal is a really useful tool during this journey as you can use it to record your reasons for wanting to fast, your specific goals, and visualizations. If you are tracking metrics, you can also use it to chart your progress in your fast and how it compares to other water fasts you may do.

5

EVERYTHING YOU NEED TO KNOW
ABOUT YOUR WATER FAST

At this point you have prepared your body and your mind for your fast, and you are about to get ready to water fast for the first time. What should you expect to happen in your body and mind while you are fasting? How long should your fast be, and what can you expect to happen at different points during your fast? In this chapter, I will guide you on the completion of a successful water fast from start to finish.

A CHANCE TO RECONNECT

As you begin your water fasting journey, consider this a time to reconnect with your body. You are going to be resetting many of your body's processes and taking yourself out of the unnatural constantly fed state that you are in right now. This is, therefore, the perfect time to build a deeper connection with your body so that, even after your fast ends, you are able to maintain an intuition about what it is that you really need to function at a high level. We spend so much time rushing through life that it is easy to ignore the small changes in our body that actually end up being signs of a deeper issue. When we take time to reconnect with our body and reestablish the connection that stress, anxiety, and modern living has all but severed, we take one of the most important steps toward good health. With the huge increase in the number of pharmaceutical interventions that are now available to us, many of us have reached the stage of answering everything our body tells us with a pill. Headaches are probably one of the most common examples of that. A headache is simply our body telling us that something is happening in our body that we need to pay attention to. It could be that we are dehydrated or stressed, or it could just be a side effect of toxins leaving our body. We simply don't take the time to investigate the cause of these signs our body gives us anymore. Instead, at the first sign of a twinge of pain between the eyes, we pop a tablet. The pain goes away, but it doesn't solve the issue that our body was raising in the first place. Gaining weight and obesity are other signals that our body gives us that we try to ignore in the wrong way. Weight gain is our body's way of telling us that something is wrong, either with the nutrition that we are consuming or at a deeper level within the systems of our body. Instead of undertaking fad diets to just reduce our weight temporarily without addressing the actual issue, water fasting helps us to reset our body so that the issue that originally caused the weight gain is addressed.

It is important to consider your fasting journey as just that—a journey, not a destination. Take the journey slowly and savor every step along the way. This is not a time to rush through, just to get to the other side. If your goal is to get through water fasting just so that you can eat again, then you are already starting with the wrong mindset. There are many things that you can learn about yourself and your body during this time if you allow yourself to.

It is vital to enter into this with the mindset that you are able to start a healing process. We are all born with the ideal and perfect system, but sadly as we get older, we don't always look after our bodies the way we should. Through water fasting, you are looking to reset a lifetime of poor eating habits and overall poor lifestyle, and that is not going to be an easy journey. Just as emotional healing from a trauma means that we have to bring all of the difficult memories to the surface to work through them before we can heal, so does physical healing mean that we are going to have to experience some uncomfortable moments in order to start the healing process. If you want an easy way to achieve this, you will have to wait until such a way is discovered because it doesn't exist yet. Nothing that is worth achieving is easy, and fasting is the same. The benefits that you will receive from fasting are definitely worth the difficulties you may experience during the early days of water fasting. You have to be willing to take it one step at a time. As you fast and feel yourself struggling with one or another part of the fast, try to take the time to interrogate yourself and find out why you are really struggling with that particular element of the fast. This deep self-interrogation could lead to great discoveries about who you are as a person and what you value. This is why it is truly important to practice water fasting when you are in a rested state and you have the ability and time to reflect on your experience and get the most out of it.

As you proceed through your fast, listen to your body and pay attention to how you are feeling. You really know your body better than anyone else, so although you will be experiencing fasting for the first time, if you begin to feel severely ill, rather play it on the safe side and halt your fast. You can always pick it up again at another time, and that is preferable to making yourself really ill.

WHAT TO DRINK AND WHAT NOT TO DRINK

Although it's called water fasting, there are other water-related beverages that you can drink during your fast as long as they contain zero calories. Any intake of calories will immediately stop your fast, so it is vital to ensure that any beverages you take in do not contain any caloric content.

Filtered water is your absolute best option for fasting. You can add a bit of Himalayan or sea salt to the water, which will help you to maintain your electrolyte levels while fasting. A depletion in electrolytes can lead to dizziness, nausea, and headaches, so if you are experiencing any of these symptoms while fasting, you can either add the salt to your water or put a pinch on the back of your tongue. You can also infuse your water with different flavors as long as they are zero calorie. You could use mint, lemon, lime, watermelon, strawberry, or even cucumber to make your water more interesting.

Ensure that you have multivitamins lined up to avoid experiencing any deficiencies and take them every day at the same time. Read the label on the multivitamins you choose to take to ensure that there are no additives which may have a calorie count. Try to avoid caffeinated drinks like black coffee and tea, as although caffeine is thought to stave off hunger, it is also an addictive toxin which will make your fast more difficult. Herbal tea is an excellent alternative as a warm drink; again, depending on the brand you choose, be sure to read the label to ensure the tea has no caloric content. Green tea is possibly one of the most beneficial warm drinks that you can consume while fasting and even when you are not fasting. There are many studies that confirm that green tea is beneficial in weight loss. Green tea contains compounds such as green tea catechins (GTC) and the most powerful of these, concerning weight loss, is epigallocatechin gallate or EGCG. The way in which GTCs aid in weight loss is rather interesting and unexpected. These catechins mimic a state in the body which is similar to our fight-or-flight mode. When we are in this mode, our body releases hormones like noradrenaline which indicate that we need to start burning energy stores at a higher rate in order to give us the strength to either fight or run away. Green tea is particularly beneficial in burning belly fat, which we know is one of the most dangerous forms of fat and also the most difficult to get rid of. A study conducted on participants who had been diagnosed with type 2 diabetes showed that the consumption of green tea helped them to reduce their waist size (reduce belly fat), even though the rest of their body weight was unchanged. This indicates that the GTCs directly target this belly fat above all other types. Another interesting impact of GTCs is that they have been shown to directly reduce levels of ghrelin in the body, thereby making us feel less hungry.

An optimum amount of water to drink, which will vary from person to person, is about 9 to 13 glasses of water. This should be consumed throughout the day to give your body time to absorb it. Drinking too much water at once can make you as ill as drinking too little water. If you feel hunger pangs become quite noticeable, drink a glass of water or two to fill your stomach up and help ease your hunger.

HOW TO DEAL WITH CHALLENGING SIDE EFFECTS

If you prepare yourself beforehand for some of the challenges you may face while fasting, you will be in a far better position to deal with them.

Initially, you may experience some lightheadedness or dizziness while fasting. This could be as a result of your body adjusting to having to use existing energy sources, and if this is the case, it will subside after a nap, which will allow your body to realign its energy usage. Dizziness may also be due to dehydration, so certainly the first thing to do when you begin to feel dizzy is drink a glass or two of water. Make sure that you add a small amount of salt to this water or a pinch on your tongue, as it may also be an electrolyte imbalance which is impacting you.

Another way that you can deal with dizziness is by sitting quietly, closing your eyes, and breathing deeply. Make sure that your in-breath and out-breath are of equal lengths so that you are ridding your lungs of all the carbon dioxide before you take in another breath of oxygen. Continue to do this for a few minutes, focusing not on your lightheadedness but rather on your breathing. Visualizations can also help to make you feel more balanced while you practice deep breathing. With your eyes closed, visualize the oxygen going into your lungs as a stream of white light that is flushing out all of the toxins and then, on the exhale, visualize yourself expelling all of those toxins into the air. This will help you to recenter your thinking on healing and not to focus on the side effects you may be experiencing. If at any time you faint or lose consciousness, stop your fast immediately and consult a doctor.

The reason that we don't recommend you carry out any strenuous acts during your water fast is because, in the initial period at least, beginner fasters are likely to feel quite weak. Your body is undergoing a major transition, and although you may not physically be working out, your cells are having the exercise session of their lives. This weakness will begin to fade and will eventually be replaced by significant energy.

The focus on water in water fasting helps to avoid many of the side effects that people practicing other forms of fasting, such as intermittent fasting (which doesn't have a focus on water consumption), may experience. Headaches, hunger, constipation, and even cravings can all be aided with the consumption of water and electrolytes through salt.

In avoiding your focus on hunger, you can chew on zero-calorie substitutes like fennel seeds or mint leaves. Adding natural hunger busters like cinnamon to your herbal tea is another good option to help stave off hunger pangs. At the root of it, hunger needs to be understood to be conquered during fasting. Hunger, similar to cravings, comes in waves and usually only lasts a few minutes at most. If you can ride out the wave, you can get past the hunger. It simply involves riding out each wave as it comes and not submitting to it. Many people actually have no idea what real hunger feels like. So many of us have bought into the societal ideal of three meals per day that we time our meals by the clock and not by when our body asks for food. Often, we don't even know what it feels like when our body asks for food because it is not our body we are listening to. By approaching your water fast as a journey of discovery, you may find it easier to deal with hunger, or what you think is hunger. Notice how different your so-called hunger alert feels on day one of your fast compared to how it feels on day three of your fast. Also, notice how quickly your body adjusts to not having food because that is its natural state. While your brain may be telling you that you are about to starve to death, your body is wiser than that. Your body understands that it is at no risk at all. It is the mental signals that we need to learn to interpret correctly so that we can tie in the wisdom of our body with the functioning of our minds and the thoughts they create. If you have developed an emotional connection to food, as many of us have without realizing it, you may experience a strange pushback from your brain in the first few days. You may have convinced your brain that food is a reward, a treat, or something you have earned, and when you don't eat, your brain wants to know why you are punishing yourself. You will eventually break this emotional connection to food. Keep reminding yourself that your water fast is your reward. What you are doing is good for you, and it is in no way a punishment. For those who are more analytical, it may be helpful to think of hunger simply as a hormone acting in your body. You know that ghrelin, the hunger hormone, is what is causing your body to feel the way it does. Instead of focusing on the actual feeling of hunger, rather focus your analytical mind, for a few minutes, on picturing how this hormone is working in your body. Acknowledge its presence, thank it for its work, and then drink water to satisfy it. If we are realistic about hunger, we know that the deep gnawing feeling we know as hunger only lasts a few seconds. One or two bites of food would make that feeling disappear completely, and that shows how negligible that feeling is. If one or two bites of food could make the feeling go away, then it is actually quite an easy feeling to ignore and move past.

Some fasting experts suggest having stevia on hand if you were a high sugar consumer prefast. Stevia is a natural sugar replacement which, in most cases, has no caloric content. This is a good way to get a little sweetness into your water without actual sugar or calorie content. Sometimes that is all that is needed to give you a little pick-me-up and urge you forward.

LIFESTYLE CHANGES

In order to get the most out of water fasting, you really need to be willing and able to make some lifestyle changes while you are fasting. I have already indicated the prefast changes that should be made in order to make your fast easier and more successful, and I have outlined the type of activities that you should focus on while you are fasting. The time during which you are fasting really needs to be a self-care period in which you listen to your body and give it what it needs in terms of rest and hydration.

It is important to avoid stress as much as possible during fasting, and if you plan to exercise, keep it to light exercises like yoga and stretching. If you start to feel really faint and drained about halfway through your fast, you can try drinking a bit of bone broth, which will provide you with salts and minerals to replenish your electrolytes. For vegetarians or vegans, instant miso soup from your local health shop will be a perfect replacement. If this is insufficient, try eating a small piece of raw fruit if absolutely necessary. Rather than push yourself to the point of really not enjoying a water fast the first time round, break early if you need to and then you can work your way up on your next fast. There has to be a first time for everything, and really, it's about gaining the experience of your first water fast so that you can build on that and gain the confidence to grow in your fasting journey.

When you start including water fasting as a regular event in your life, it is a good idea to schedule it sometime in advance so that you can allocate your preparation time and really set yourself up for success. While water fasting is a very individual exercise, encouragement and bonding with others can be beneficial, especially when you are new to water fasting. There are quite a few online forums, especially on social media, in which water fasting is a hot topic. While you may find great support on such forums, also ensure that you research and verify any information that is provided by members of the public.

Curiosity can be a very rewarding trait, and your water fasting journey is a great time to develop curiosity about your body and its response to certain conditions. Rather than relying on the studies of others, use your water fasting journey to create some of your own research and, in so doing, learn more about how your body works. You can track various metrics to measure your progress and response along the way. By doing this, you can also have peace of mind about what is happening in your body. Some of the metrics you can consider tracking include:

- ketones
- pH balance
- cholesterol
- liver function
- iron levels
- vitamin D levels
- body measurements
- body fat percentage
- weight
- muscle mass percentage
- body water percentage

You don't need to go to the doctor every time you want to test one of these metrics. You can purchase home testing kits for all of the above-mentioned metrics online to track your progress in the comfort of your own home. To get good data, start tracking these metrics before you even begin your preparation phase. You can record these on a computer or in a notebook. If you are conducting an initial 24-hour fast, test yourself before you start your preparation, then once in the middle of your fast, once after your postfast period, and wait a few days after you resume your normal eating routine and test yourself again. In this way, you don't need to guess as to the difference that water fasting is having on your body or rely on how you feel. You can have facts in number form right in front of you. While each individual will differ, the following are the average acceptable ranges for the metrics you may test:

- Ketones: you will be in ketosis if your reading is 1.5 to 3.0 mmol/l
- pH balance: normal pH level of the human body is 7.40
- Cholesterol: LDL cholesterol levels should be less than 100mg/dL
- Liver function: AST liver function is normal at 10-40 units per liter, and ALT liver function is normal at 7-56 per liter
- Iron levels: 35.5-44.9%
- Vitamin D levels: 20-50 ng/mL
- Body measurements: per individual
- Body fat percentage: 21-33% in women and 8-19% in men
- Weight: per individual
- Muscle mass percentage: this is highly dependent on age and gender, but in general, a good range is between 30.4 and 35.1% for women and between 39.4 and 44% for men
- Body water percentage: 45-65%

By measuring these metrics, you can also see what works for you as an individual and what doesn't. If you are unsure about what might break your fast and you are getting conflicting information in your research, test it out by measuring your ketones before and after.

By really drilling down into these measurable metrics, you will be able to gain a factual basis for your standpoint on water fasting. If the tests and readings all seem a bit overwhelming, choose the ones that will align best with your goals. If you are trying to lose weight, you will want to know if you are going into fat burning so make testing your ketones a priority.

6

THE POSTFAST PERIOD

J ust as the way in which you start your fast and the things you do while you are fasting are important, the way you end your fast is vital. By ending your fast in the wrong way, you can actually undo a lot of the good you have done, and in the worst-case scenario, you can make yourself ill. Breaking your water fast is almost a reverse of the actions you took when you started your fast, and it encourages a seamless transition back into your normal routine. The longer you have fasted for, the more important a gradual breaking of the fast becomes.

In one of the most common religious fasts, the Muslim fast of Ramadan, it has been noted that followers commonly break their fast with a small meal. They will then attend a prayer service for the evening and only after they return will they enjoy a full meal. This type of fasting is very different from water fasting and is more in line with intermittent fasting, but the slow breaking of the fast is applicable even here and outlines its importance. In research that has been undertaken around followers of the Ramadan fast, those who do not break their fast in such a way, and instead launch into a huge meal to break their fast, report feeling ill, gaining weight, and experiencing severe indigestion. Due to the fact that water fasting is so much more intense than this type of religious fasting and, in most cases, much longer, the breaking of the fast becomes all the more important.

Another common mistake is thinking that as soon as your water fast ends, you can immediately start with strenuous activity and resume your normal routine immediately. Just as your body needs time to ease into water fasting, it also needs time to ease out.

RESTARTING YOUR DIGESTIVE SYSTEM

Depending on how long you have water fasted for on this occasion, you must be consciously aware of the fact that you have essentially halted your digestive process for the entire time that you have been fasting. The production of gastric juices has mostly stopped, and your digestive system is going to be sluggish to begin with. Consider a vehicle that has been standing for a long time. You wouldn't jump in, rev the engine ferociously, and immediately race off down the road, would you? Instead, you would start the engine and let it run for a while, allowing it to heat up before racing away with it. By the same token, your digestive system must be restarted slowly. If you immediately flood your digestive system with a huge amount of foods that are difficult to digest, it is almost always going to struggle to digest that food properly.

When you break a fast, you are rebuilding your digestive system, which includes your gut and stomach lining. Breaking a fast too quickly will result in toxins being created in your body, and you will have wasted the time you spent fasting. A baby does not come out of the womb munching down on a cheeseburger and fries. We start infants off with a liquid diet and slowly work them up to solids. A similar process applies to coming out of a fast.

Ideally, break your fast with a glass of fruit juice, preferably one that you have prepared at home so that you avoid the high amounts of sugar that are often in store-bought juices. Orange and lime juice are good options, and you can add a spoonful of honey to it if necessary. A light vegetable soup or a glass of coconut water is also a good way to break your fast, with the latter containing a huge amount of beneficial electrolytes. Wait about half an hour for this initial consumption to digest and see how you feel. If you feel a little ill, wait a bit longer to move on to the next step. If you feel fine, you can move onto a fruit smoothie. Again, give your body time to digest this smoothie. Preferably, don't spend this time focused on food and thinking about what you are going to eat next. Instead, continue with a low-stress activity and try to keep your mind off food. In a few hours, if you are feeling well and your stomach is not bloated or uncomfortable, you can eat a small amount of fermented food such as sauerkraut or a source of healthy fat like avocado. Although kefir is a very popular fermented food, it is not good for breaking a water fast as it is dairy based in origin and, therefore, more difficult to digest.

Keep in mind that you need to apply as much discipline in breaking your fast as you did in your preparation and during your water fast. The general rule is that your postfast recovery should be the same number of days over which your fast lasted. If you fasted for 24 hours, then you should not eat a full meal until 24 hours after ending your fast. This also depends on the individual. If you are an otherwise healthy individual with a normally strong digestive system, you could break your fast a bit quicker, but if you suffer from health conditions and usually have a sluggish digestive system, you may want to take it even slower. As with all other stages of a water fast, listen to your body and take it slow.

It is important not to let your guard down at the point of breaking your fast. You have done such good work so far and worked hard to give your body this natural reset, so it would be a pity to see all of that hard work go to waste by allowing yourself to slip back into your normal routine immediately. Guard your mental and emotional state at this time, as well, as your brain will likely be telling you to go back to your usual food routine. It is important to consider how good your normal routine was to begin with. One of the most exciting parts about fasting is that you have essentially wiped your nutritional slate clean. If you have ever wanted to eat a better diet, now is the time to do so. If you have been wanting to switch over to a plant-based diet, for instance, your body and mind are now in the prime state to make that change. Consider this as you ease back into eating as your "normal" routine is very likely not the best to revert back to. In terms of exercise, if your usual routine involves strenuous exercise, don't get back into this for at least a week after you have resumed normal eating. Instead practice yoga, stretch, and take short walks. Just as you build up your eating, you should also build up the exercise and activity you do, slowly and progressively to avoid overexerting yourself.

When we return to eating after a fast, there is a significant possibility of reactive weight gain if we immediately return to a diet of processed and unhealthy foods. It would be unfortunate to work hard during a fast to cleanse your body and possibly lose weight only to pick up additional weight after a water fast simply because you have gone back to an unhealthy diet.

SAMPLE FAST-BREAKING DAY

How you break your water fast is very important and, as such, it is important to remove any confusion about exactly what you should eat and when during your postfast period. As an example of how a fast should be broken, I will lay out an eating guide which you can use in order to break your fast. This guide will work on the presumption that you have undertaken a 72-hour (3-day) fast, but if you have only fasted for 24 hours, you can still apply the same idea, just over a shorter period. Feel free to switch up the ingredients to items that you are able to get or that are affordable for you.

Day One

This is the first day of eating after your fast. Your digestive system is very sensitive on this day, and it is important to take it slow and ensure you don't overdo it. On this day, you will not take in any solid food. Start with a glass of fruit juice, a small cup of vegetable soup, bone broth, or coconut water. Do not take in any dairy product on this day as they are very difficult to digest and will disturb your digestive system. Essentially, what you want to eat today is just one step up from water—a liquid that contains some calories but preferably more nutrients.

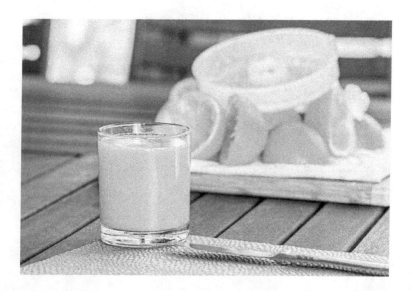

Don't jump into any strenuous activities right away either. Give your body time to adjust to the fact that you are feeding it again. Your digestive system is slowly starting up. Consume your food slowly at all times. With today's liquid diet, sip slowly and give the body time to move the liquid down to your stomach before taking another sip. Gulping down your first liquid meal is going to make you feel rather ill, and you will enjoy it far more if you consume it slowly.

Day Two

Today you can move on to light and easily digested solids. Good options for today would include papaya, avocado, watermelon, cantaloupe, and ripe banana. Have some of these fruits in the morning and pay attention to how your digestive system reacts. This will be a good indication of whether you are moving too fast. If you feel ill or uncomfortable or begin to vomit when you first take in solid foods, revert back to liquid for another day as your digestive system needs more time to adjust. If you ingest these fruits in the morning or early afternoon and feel well, you can prepare a plate of boiled vegetables as an early dinner. Potato is an easily digestible starch vegetable for this meal but eat only a small portion. Cruciferous vegetables like broccoli, cauliflower, and brussels sprouts are difficult to digest, so they should be avoided. Vegetables that are easy to digest include yellow squash, pumpkin, spinach, beets, green beans, and carrots. Don't eat too late in the day when you are breaking your fast as our metabolism naturally slows down when we sleep, and you want to ensure that you have digested your food properly before you go to sleep.

Remember to chew your food really well so that you help your digestive system to get going again. In general, most people do not chew their food sufficiently and also eat far too quickly. This results in us consuming more food than we need because we are missing the full signal in our brains. It also results in indigestion, which is almost like traffic congestion for your digestive system. If you let everything in at once, your body doesn't have time to move it down to your stomach, and you will end up feeling like half your meal is stuck in your esophagus.

Day Three

Today you can have your first solid meal. It is preferable to only eat one such meal in the day, and the best time is around midday to allow for full digestion. Keep your portions small and avoid any processed foods. Don't include any spice in your food and try to stick to foods like rice, wheat, or oats. An excellent option would be a bowl of cooked oats with ripe banana. Other good options include eggs, avocado, nuts, and spinach. Stick to soft foods for a while and definitely avoid meat for as long as you can after you have completed your fast.

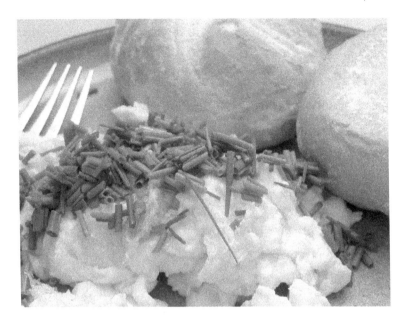

For the rest of the day, continue with fruit juices, smoothies, and boiled vegetables. Pay close attention to how you are feeling after you eat this meal both physically and emotionally. If you feel that you have moved too quickly, revert back to day one or two and start again. You literally cannot move too slowly in breaking your fast. While raw foods might sound healthier, they are also more difficult to digest, and it's not recommended within your immediate postfast period. Another ideal first meal may be a scrambled egg with soft cooked vegetables and a few cubes of avocado.

Day Four Onward

Slowly increase your number of meals and portions until you are eating a well-rounded, balanced diet again. Again, try to use this period of readjustment to make changes to your diet that you have always wanted to. This period is also very important in understanding the hidden obsessions with foods that may exist in our psyche. By taking this breaking of fast slowly, you can pay attention, not just to your physical body but also to what is happening in your mind as you reintroduce food into your routine. Remember to chew properly and don't eat too quickly. By doing this, you will also find that you feel fuller quicker as you give your body time to recognize that it is receiving food and register fullness.

Once you have completed your fast, consider what foods you really missed. If you didn't particularly miss eating meat, for instance, this might be the ideal time to cut it out entirely. While lean meat is a good source of protein in moderation, when eaten too often it can cause a myriad of health issues. In increasing the amount of fruit and vegetables that you eat, keep in mind that it doesn't have to be fresh to be healthy. In the past frozen fruit and vegetables held only a small portion of the nutrients that the fresh option did. Freezing technology in the food industry has grown significantly, though, and today, there are just as many nutrients in the frozen option. Fruit can also be kept frozen for smoothies, which are not just easy on the digestive system but a great way to include a wide variety of fruits and vegetables in your diet.

When restructuring your postfast diet, stay away from low-fat products. This may sound counterintuitive, but the low-fat fad that once swept the food market has started to make way for full-fat options again as people have realized the deception behind the low-fat label. When manufacturers make products "low-fat," they have to include something else in the product to make up for the missing fat, and what they usually include is carbohydrates. If you carefully compare the label of a low-fat yogurt, for example, compared to a full-fat or medium-fat product, you will see that the carbohydrate level on the low-fat option is far higher. These are also not good carbohydrates that are easily digested by your body; they are refined carbohydrates.

Another small adjustment that you can make to your diet which will have a big impact is to use fresh herbs in your cooking. Buy bunches of fresh herbs and store them in your fridge with the stems in a glass of water. In this way, you can keep them fresh for up to two weeks and just snip off what you would like as you go. Fresh herbs are a fantastic source of natural medicinal properties. At the same time, keep a head of ginger and a bulb of turmeric root in your freezer for the same reason. These can be grated from frozen into food. The following are some examples of healthy herbs and spices that you should use more often in cooking:

- Turmeric: excellent in curries and a powerful anti-inflammatory when paired with a fat like coconut oil and black pepper.
- Cinnamon: helps to reduce blood sugar levels, stave off hunger, and has a powerful antidiabetic effect.

- Sage: has been used to great effect in research trials with Alzheimer's Disease patients and helps to improve brain function and memory.
- Peppermint: helps to relieve pain from irritable bowel syndrome and aids in treating nausea.
- Basil: excellent in Italian dishes and also helps fight infections and boost immunity.
- Cayenne pepper: helps to reduce appetite and has cancer-fighting properties.
- Ginger: also fabulous in curries and can treat nausea and has anti-inflammatory properties.
- Fenugreek: has beneficial effects in leveling out blood sugar.
- Rosemary: prevents nasal congestion and allergies
- Garlic: contains allicin which combats illness and improves heart health. (Tip: when cooking with fresh garlic, don't cut and cook immediately. Peel the clove and then crush and allow to sit for a few minutes before cooking. This gives the allicin time to build up to its highest levels.)

It is important to understand the difference in various fats as well, as the word has become synonymous with something bad in the last few decades, and that is really not the case. We need fats in our diet, but we need the right fats. There are two types of fats in general: saturated and unsaturated fats. Saturated fats are bad for us. They are found in processed meats and junk food. Unsaturated fats are good for us and we need them. An example of this is omega-3 that is found in wild-caught salmon. It is just as unhealthy to cut out all of the good fats in our diet as it is to include too many bad fats. From a cooking oil perspective, plant-based oils are generally unsaturated except for the tropical oils like coconut and palm oil.

One of the greatest things about water fasting is that it doesn't require a range of expensive and exotic foods in order to accomplish the goal. Many of the fad diets we see call for some of the wildest ingredients and wilder still, is what those ingredients cost. Water fasting is accessible to everyone because it doesn't cost anything, and you will actually end up saving money because you won't be eating during your fast. Feel free to structure your postfast eating to food available in your region and that suits your budget. We spend a lot of time thinking about, preparing, and eating food, and you will likely be pleasantly surprised by how much time and money you save when you fast.

REFEEDING SYNDROME

A slow reintroduction of food into the system after water fasting is so vital as there is a specific syndrome that can develop if a person who has experienced an extended period without food suddenly gorges on huge amounts of solid food. While this syndrome is far more common in people who have suffered from eating disorders or who have not voluntarily stopped eating, it is important to understand what the syndrome entails. The slow progression into and out of a water fast is the difference between a healthy reset of your digestive system and other body processes and a possibly damaging experience.

Refeeding syndrome is seen when food is too quickly reintroduced to people who have experienced an absence of nutrition for a protracted period. It is characterized by the sudden production of glycogen, protein, and fat, which leads to low concentrations of minerals such as phosphorus, magnesium, and potassium in the blood. The pulmonary and cardiac systems can be affected, and the person may even experience neurological symptoms. When insulin production is forced to resume in the body at an accelerated rate, the increase of the synthesis of macronutrients uses up the minimal mineral stores far too quickly, and when these stores are so quickly depleted, it can have devastating effects on the body.

While refeeding syndrome is extremely rare in those coming out of water fasting, it is important to understand the impact that it can have on the body so that exceptional emphasis is placed on the postfast period.

7

OTHER COMMON QUESTIONS ABOUT WATER FASTING

I n this chapter, I will answer some of the questions that you still may have around water fasting that have not yet been addressed. As water fasting has become more popular, several myths have sprung up around the practice, and it is important to address those. By fully educating yourself around water fasting and entering into the practice with no doubts or questions, you can experience a safe and beneficial fast.

How Long Can I Fast For?

The human body can go for about a month without food. Such a period for fasting is neither necessary nor healthy, though, as you can glean the same benefits from shorter periods. The "slow and steady" approach cannot be emphasized enough. There is no benefit for a first-time faster to enter into a 7-day fast. Not only will you likely fail, but it will be a very difficult and uncomfortable experience. If you have never fasted before, start with 24 hours or less. Once you have achieved a full 24-hour water fast and you feel comfortable and well, you can consider working your way up. Eventually you could build yourself up to 7 to 14 days of water fasting if your lifestyle allows for this. Keep in mind that the period that you choose to actually fast in must be multiplied by three in order to calculate how much time you actually need for the prefast and postfast activities. For an active, relatively healthy person, a 72-hour fast once per month is ideal. Studies have also shown that age can impact the length for which you can safely fast. The general rule of thumb is that the higher your nutritional needs at a particular stage of life, the shorter your fast should be. It is for this reason that children under the age of 18 should not fast at all as they need high levels of nutrition to grow. Young adults are often still in bone and brain development and can handle shorter fasts. The optimum age group to start longer fasting is around 40. At this age, your nutritional requirements are lower, and you are able to handle going without food for longer periods. As we age, we can fast for even longer periods. If you suffer from health conditions or you are overweight, you can consider going for a longer fast on several occasions throughout the year, but you should always consult a doctor first.

Why Do I Experience Unpleasant Side Effects While Fasting?

The irony of toxins is that they feel great going in and horrendous coming out. Processed and junk food tastes delicious, smoking is a pleasurable addiction for some, and alcohol consumption seems fun and casual while you are doing it. The toxins that these things create in our body, though, are so bad for us that when we undergo a process like water fasting to rid our bodies of them, we tend to feel ill while it's happening. The process of healing and detoxification can, unfortunately, be uncomfortable, but it is not only very necessary but highly beneficial in the long run. Symptoms of detoxification during a water fast can include dizziness, nausea, diarrhea, and skin breakouts or a change in skin composition. While these side effects are not pleasant, they should never make you feel violently ill or lose consciousness. Detoxification from severe toxins like hard drugs is done under medical supervision only because it is a very dangerous process. If you feel like your body is reacting very severely to a normal detoxification process while water fasting, you should stop immediately and see a doctor.

Will I Lose Muscle Mass When I Fast?

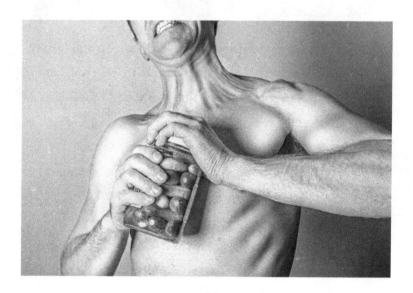

The short answer to this question is when done correctly water fasting should never cause the loss of muscle mass. Losing muscle mass is certainly not an aim of water fasting, and it is not beneficial to our body. When we water fast, we aim to first work through our glucose stores and then move onto our fat deposits. Depending on the length of your fast, most of your weight loss will come from water weight, and while you will feel leaner, there will be no reduction in your muscle mass. Fasting actually promotes the production of human growth hormone which plays a significant role in the production of muscle tissue. The higher levels of human growth hormone in your blood will also work to protect your muscles from wastage.

Will I Regain the Weight I Lost After My Fast Ends?

The possibility of regaining weight depends on the type of weight you have lost while water fasting. If you have done a 24-hour fast, then you have likely lost water weight, and this will be regained when you resume your normal food consumption. Research shows that you may lose up to two pounds per day during a 24-hour to 72-hour fast, but much of the initial weight will be water weight. If you have moved past your glucose stores and started burning fat, however, that weight loss can be maintained with the correct postfast activities. If you break your fast correctly and continue to eat a healthy, balanced diet when your fasting is complete, you have a far greater chance of maintaining your weight loss. Remember that in your few initial fasts, weight loss should not be the main goal. Instead, you should be focused on getting your body used to water fasting so that you can undertake longer fasts in which you will lose more weight. You are also resetting your digestive system and food consumption habits during fasting, so while you may not lose a huge amount of weight during the actual fast, the changes in your body and lifestyle thereafter could aid in additional weight loss.

How Can I Deal With Headaches While Fasting?

Headaches experienced during water fasting can be a result of a wide variety of causes. The most common reason you develop headaches while fasting is due to dehydration, and this is a sign that you have not increased your water consumption enough to make up for the fluid that you would usually get from food. In order to remove toxins, your body needs water, and if there is insufficient water available to get rid of the level of toxins that need to be expelled, they will start to build up in your system. This build will cause, among other symptoms, headaches. If you start to feel a headache building, immediately drink one or two glasses of water. If this is indeed the cause of your headache, the pain will start to ease within half an hour. If you do not receive relief from drinking water, you can also try putting a pinch of salt on the back of your tongue. This will help to replenish your electrolytes. Peppermint oil is known to provide relief for headaches, and this is certainly something you should try. Peppermint oil can be used by placing a few drops in your bath. You can also pour hot water into a bowl, add a few drops of peppermint oil to the water, cover your head and the bowl with a towel, and inhale and exhale deeply into the steam. Do this for about two minutes. You could also make peppermint tea by steeping peppermint leaves in hot water for a few minutes. Do not ingest peppermint essential oil unless it is food grade and, even then, only if it is zero calorie. When fasting, medication for headaches should always be a last resort. It is not good to take medication on an empty stomach, and if you develop a headache or migraine to such an extent that you cannot relieve it with any of the aforementioned tips or a nap, you may want to consider ending your fast instead and trying again at a later stage.

What Can I Do About Heartburn While Fasting?

In the initial stages of your fast, you may experience heartburn as your stomach hasn't entirely stopped producing gastric acids yet, but it also doesn't have any food to work on. This may result in a burning sensation in your chest or near your diaphragm. For some people this may be the first time they have experienced heartburn, and it could be a rather alarming sensation. Warm water works well to reduce heartburn. To help during the day, start the morning off with a glass of warm water, which should be slowly sipped and not gulped all at once. It may also help to take a nap while keeping your head elevated and your upper body propped up.

If you suffer from severe heartburn or gastroesophageal reflux disorder, you may want to consider intermittent rather than water fasting as when the stomach is empty and continues to make stomach acid for long periods, this can lead to a worsening of the condition.

What Could Happen to My Bowel Movements While I Am Fasting?

The impact of water fasting on bowel movements is quite an individual experience. You may experience constipation, you may experience no need to have a bowel movement at all, or you may experience diarrhea. All of these instances are normal and depend on how you have prepared your body for the fast as well as how many toxins you need to remove from your body. Your bowel movement is one of the ways that your body uses to remove waste products and toxins from your food that are left over after food has been digested. It stands to reason that if you are not taking in any food, then there is nothing to come out, so if you don't feel the need to have a bowel movement at all, you needn't be concerned. If you ordinarily are not very regular or you haven't prepared very well in the run-up to your fast, then you may find that you become constipated as you may still have some fecal matter left in your bowel when you start fasting, and due to the changes in your digestive system, your body struggles to get that out. In this case, try to increase your water intake slightly as this can help you to move your bowels. If constipation becomes painful or very uncomfortable, you can try using a mild laxative suppository after consulting a doctor. In some cases, your body will use your bowel to cleanse itself of all the toxins it is cleaning out, and you may experience diarrhea. The stool in this case may be strange in color or odor, but you should not be alarmed unless you see any blood in your stool. If you do develop diarrhea, be sure to increase your water intake as you will be losing a lot of water with your stool which will need to be replenished to avoid developing dehydration.

How Often Can I Do a Water Fast?

Beginners can fast for 24 hours once per week but keep in mind that this involves an extra two days—one before and one after—for prefast and postfast activities. If you are able to allocate three days per week to the type of environment that it takes to water fast properly, then you can do that. You could elect to fast every second weekend as you will likely not be working or attending college at that time, and you can undertake a 24-hour fast properly. Once you feel that you are getting used to fasting and 24 hours is becoming relatively easy to accomplish, you can not only start to increase the period that you fast but also increase the gap in between fasts. So, as your next level up, for instance, you could do a three-day fast once per month or once every two months. As water fasting becomes part of your lifestyle, you will start to feel when your body needs to fast again, and you can then find an appropriate period of time in your schedule to do so. If you are experiencing a great deal of stress but also feel like your body needs a water fast, rather try an intermittent fast or simply eat clean and whole foods instead of conducting a proper water fast. When the period of stress has passed, then you can water fast again. There is no set schedule for the number of times you should fast per week, month, or year as every individual is different. In all cases, start small and work your way up. You will get great benefit from any amount of fasting, and studies show that just one 24-hour period of fasting per month can reduce your risk of heart attack by up to 40% (Water Fasting, 2020).

Is Water Fasting Safe for Women?

Much has been said about the delicate balance of various hormones in a woman's body and the possibility that fasting of any nature could put these out of balance. There is no scientific evidence to prove that water fasting has any negative impact on the sex hormones in a woman's body. In fact, water fasting is ideal for menopausal and postmenopausal women as it helps to balance out the levels of estrogen in their body and increase the levels of hormones which naturally start to decrease with age, including human growth hormone and brain-derived neurotrophic factor. Women who are trying to conceive, already pregnant, or breastfeeding should not practice water fasting until they have moved through this time. It is also probably not advisable for women to water fast at the same time as their menstrual period. This has nothing to do with hormone levels, though, and it is more a matter of convenience and comfort. Women can already feel rather unwell during their menstrual period so to add the pressure of fasting onto that would not be a good idea. Studies have shown that women actually tend to do slightly better on water fasts than men because their energy requirements are smaller.

Why Do I Feel Bloated When I Start Eating Again?

If you experience bloating when you start eating again after a fast, then you have likely started with solids too quickly. As each digestive system is different, even if you only did a 24-hour fast and started eating solids within the recommended 24-hour period after your fast, it may simply be too soon for your body. Go back to juices and smoothies and slowly work your way back up to solid food.

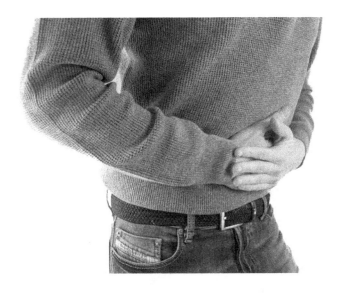

The types of food you eat, in general, can also add to bloating, but that is not always a bad thing. Some foods are not broken down by gastric acid; instead, they sit in your gut and are fermented by your gut bacteria. This fermentation process releases gases which can cause bloating and flatulence, but this process is actually very good for your gut. By providing your gut bacteria with foods that contain resistant starches such as beans and cruciferous vegetables, you are giving your bacteria a bit of exercise which helps to strengthen them. Your body also absorbs nutrients better through this fermentation process.

What Can I Do About Bad Breath While Fasting?

You may experience a reaction to fasting which is commonly referred to as "detox tongue." Basically, it is a build-up of white substance on the tongue which is a part of the detoxification process. Not everyone gets this side effect, but for those who do, it can be quite annoying. Other than brushing your teeth frequently and using a tongue scraper, you can also chew on mint leaves or gargle with a diluted solution of food-grade hydrogen peroxide. Be careful with store-bought mouthwash as it can contain hidden calories. Besides the accumulation of toxins on the tongue, a bad taste in your mouth or bad breath can also be caused by the larger quantity of ketones in your system. People who practice a Keto diet will be familiar with the fruity smell of the breath which is called Keto breath. This happens when we fast, too, as our ketone level increases. The best ways around this, without breaking our fast, is to brush your teeth regularly and increase your intake of water.

My Family is Concerned—How Can I Convince Them?

When people don't understand something, they tend to fear it. So, your best bet is to share the facts with them. If they are open minded, the research and data that are presented in this book and in other resources should allay their fears. Sometimes people just don't want to be convinced, though, and that's okay. If you are over the age of 18 (which you should be to water fast anyway), you don't need anyone's permission to try something new for your health. Family members or friends who are skeptical beforehand will likely be less so when they see the results at the end of your water fast. Family members who live with you are probably concerned about what your practice of fasting will mean for them. In such a case, be clear that all you need from them is to not purposefully make it more difficult for you. Explain that you do not expect them to join in water fasting and that they are more than welcome to continue with life as normal. You may want to point out the benefits that your water fasting will bring for them too. You will have more energy, you will be healthier, and you will live longer. These are all things that any loving family member or friend should value.

Can I Brush My Teeth While Fasting?

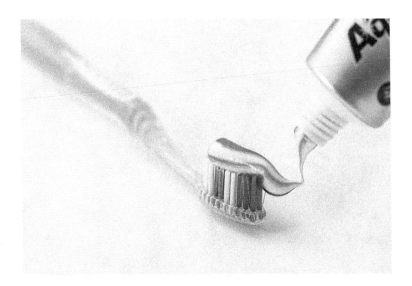

The question of whether brushing your teeth and the possible intake of a small amount of toothpaste would break the fast is often raised. Even though you are not eating, it is still a good idea to continue with your oral hygiene as you may be collecting toxins on your tongue while you sleep resulting in an unpleasant taste in your mouth as well as a bit of bad breath. Depending on the brand of your toothpaste and what it contains, there is a very good chance that it will not break your fast. Read the ingredients to be sure, but the small amount of toothpaste that you may ingest while brushing will likely have almost no effect on insulin levels.

CONCLUSION

For millions of years, humans ate when they had access to food. Sometimes that would be once a week, and sometimes that would be once a month. It's only been in the last few centuries, since the agricultural revolution, that we really started to build the idea of a constantly fed society. Of course, there have been significant benefits to this change. We no longer die of hunger, we don't suffer from undernutrition as much as we used to, and many nutrition-based diseases, like scurvy, have been almost completely eliminated. We are also very different in body structure now, and our energy needs are significantly different. These differences in lifestyle, though, do not account for the enormous difference in the way we eat. There has been a significant downside to this eat-on-demand culture, and now, the world's greatest nutrition-based problems are overnutrition and obesity.

As a result of this increase in obesity and the chronic illnesses which have come with it, we have seen a corresponding marked increase in the number of "quick-fix" solution fad diets. The problem with these fad diets is that they have very little basis in science, and they also do not have much social proof in terms of members of the public who have followed the diet and can say that 20 years later for instance, they've had no negative effects from it. The other problem with these diets is that all they do is help you lose weight—there are no other health benefits. Fasting, and in particular, water fasting, is the only overall weight loss and health regimen that has thousands of years of social proof. It is also the only one with significant clinical studies having been conducted which provide data to support its claimed benefits.

Despite all of these phenomenal benefits and historical significance, water fasting is not for everyone. In this book, I have clearly expressed the situations and circumstances under which water fasting is not the ideal practice. Should you have any doubts about whether water fasting would be good for you, please consult your doctor before making the decision.

I wrote this book because water fasting made an enormous difference in my life, and I wanted to share not just my experience but also the knowledge that I have gained through my studies and my patients' fasting experiences. Knowledge and research is absolutely key if you are considering water fasting because if you don't follow the correct procedures, you can not only make yourself rather ill but you may also waste your time as you could undo any benefits you gained during your fasting period. This book has covered the water fasting journey from beginning to end, providing you with the necessities for prefast preparation, the experience you can expect from the actual fasting period, as well as how to safely end your fast.

As transparency is vital in matters of health, I have also provided you with details of the clinical studies in which many of the benefits of water fasting have been proven. The links to these studies are contained in the references section, and I encourage you to view those studies yourself and also to do further research, if required, until you feel satisfied that you have done due diligence in researching the practice of water fasting.

Water fasting is not a quick-fix solution. It is a lifestyle, and once you immerse yourself in it, it becomes a phenomenal tool for improving your health both physically and mentally. I think that one of the reasons that I connected so deeply with water fasting—and I have no doubt that you will too—is that it truly is a holistic regimen. When I undertake a water fast, I don't just come out the other side a few pounds lighter. I come out rejuvenated in every way. I am a really curious person, and because I struggled so much with my health in my youth, I probably find it more interesting than many others do, to understand exactly how my body works.

In order to really gain the full array of benefits from water fasting, it is important to set time aside for the practice. It's really not something that you want to squeeze in between work and socializing, for instance. The true healing from water fasting happens when you allow yourself to simply be and provide yourself with space to recover from the difficulties of life and expel the toxins from your body that have built up over the years.

If I think about how much money the anti-ageing industry is worth—the creams, the potions, the "magic" elixirs—it is quite amazing to think that the true secret to real cellular-level anti-ageing has always been inside us, and it's free! I am excited to see what the medical community does with the revelations that have recently been made around autophagy. Its applications in disease prevention and treatment are almost endless. The most wonderful thing about the discovery of this process and its applications in our body is that we don't have to wait for permission to use it. The process has always belonged to us, and now we know how to trigger it so that no matter what our age, through water fasting we can benefit from the renewal properties of autophagy. The knowledge that we gain in learning about autophagy and water fasting and its benefits is really empowering. Most of us dread old age as we have been made to believe that we have no choice but to tumble down into a pit of illness and health difficulties. Along with that, we have been made to believe that we have no control over the fact that we will lose our cognitive abilities as we age. For some, that thought is more frightening than any other. With the knowledge we have gained in the arena of ageing in the last few years, though, we now realize that this inevitable doom of old age is simply not accurate. We can control how we age to a great extent, and we don't have to resign ourselves to suffering as we get older. By using water fasting to trigger autophagy in our body, we can make every effort to prevent chronic disease, obesity, and premature death. We just have to be willing to put in a bit of work and commitment.

As we near the end of the book, I would like to request that if the experience and knowledge that I have shared with you in *Water Fasting: How to Lose Weight Fast, Increase Mental Clarity, Heal Your Body, & Activate Autophagy With Water Fasting*, has been beneficial to you, that you pass this knowledge on too. The best way to do this is by giving the book a positive review on Amazon so that others can find the book and benefit from it too. There is truly no greater feeling than knowing that you have helped another human being to avoid the difficulties that you may have experienced. It's why I wrote this book, and it's why I am asking you to share this book. In your reviews, I would also love to hear about your water fasting experience so that we can learn and grow from the journeys of others.

Most importantly, as you start your water fasting journey, I hope that your experience will be as beneficial as mine was. We all have regrets, on occasion, about things we wish we could have done differently, especially from a health perspective. Water fasting is your chance to correct those missteps. It's a reset on our digestive system, and to a large extent, on our lifestyle. This practice is not just about losing weight. It is about using the processes that already exist in our body to greater effect by returning our way of eating to a more natural form.

If you wish to enjoy a long and healthy life free from disease, and to keep your mind sharp and focused throughout, water fasting really is your best bet. It is not a magic pill or a wave of a wand, though, and it will take work and commitment from you. The fact that you have sourced, purchased, and finished reading this book, though, shows an immense drive already. The great sense of achievement that you will experience after your first water fast is phenomenal. As you end each water fast, it is just the beginning of a new season for your body, and as you end this book, your journey begins.

DOWNLOAD YOUR FREE CHEAT SHEET

(<u>Don't</u> start fasting before you've consulted this cheat sheet...)

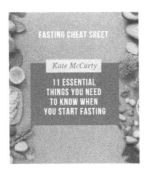

This cheat sheet includes:

- 11 things to know and to do while you are fasting.
- Why you need to know those things to start successfully.
- These things will make the process easier and more enjoyable.

The last thing I want is that the fasting process will be uncomfortable.

To receive your fasting cheat sheet, scan this QR code:

REFERENCES

30-Minute Coconut Curry. (n.d.). Retrieved from https:// minimalistbaker.com/30-minute-coconut-curry/ #_a5y_p=1531167

Allaf , M., Elghazaly , H., Mohamed , O. G., Fareen , F. K., Zaman , S., Salmasi , A. M., ... Dehghan, A. (2019). Intermittent fasting for the prevention of cardiovascular disease. Retrieved from https://www.cochranelibrary.com/cdsr/doi/10.1002/ 14651858.CD013496/full

Anton, S. D., Moehl, K., Donahoo, W., & Marosi, K. (2017). Flipping the Metabolic Switch: Understanding and Applying the Health Benefits of Fasting: Flipping the Metabolic Switch. Retrieved from https://www.researchgate.net/ publication/320733870_Flipping_the_Metabolic_Switch_Under

standing_and_Applying_the_Health_Benefits_of_Fasting_Flippi
ng_the_Metabolic_Switch

Antoni, R., Johnston, K. L., Collins, A. L., & Robertson, M. D. (2014). The Effects of Intermittent Energy Restriction on Indices of Cardiometabolic Health. Retrieved from https://ibimapublishing.com/articles/ENDO/2014/459119/

Antunes, F., Erustes, A. G., Costa, A. J., Nascimento, A. C., Bincoletto, C., Ureshino, R. P., ... Smaili, S. S. (2018). Autophagy and intermittent fasting: the connection for cancer therapy? Retrieved from https://www.ncbi.nlm.nih.gov/pmc/articles/PMC6257056/

Arnason, T. G., Bowen, M. W., & Mansell, K. D. (2017). Effects of intermittent fasting on health markers in those with type 2 diabetes: A pilot study. Retrieved from https://www.ncbi.nlm.nih.gov/pubmed/28465792

Azevedo, F. R. de, Ikeoka, D., & Caramelli, B. (2013). Effects of intermittent fasting on metabolism in men. Retrieved from https://www.sciencedirect.com/science/article/pii/S0104423013000213

Barnosky, A. R., Hoddy, K. K., Unterman, T. G., & Varady, K. A. (2014). Intermittent fasting vs daily calorie restriction for type 2 diabetes prevention: a review of human findings. Retrieved from https://www.ncbi.nlm.nih.gov/pubmed/24993615

Barnosky, A. R., Hoddy, K. K., Unterman, T. G., & Varady, K. A. (2014). Intermittent fasting vs daily calorie restriction for type 2 diabetes prevention: a review of human findings. Retrieved from https://www.sciencedirect.com/science/article/pii/S193152441400200X

Bauersfeld, S. P., Kessler, C. S., Wischnewsky, M., Jaensch, A., Steckhan, N., Stange, R., ... Michalsen, A. (2018). The effects of short-term fasting on quality of life and tolerance to chemotherapy in patients with breast and ovarian cancer: a randomized cross-over pilot study. Retrieved from https://bmccancer. biomedcentral.com/articles/10.1186/s12885-018-4353-2

Baum, I. (2019). What Is the OMAD Diet? Everything You Need to Know About This Extreme Intermittent Fasting Weight-Loss Plan. Retrieved from https://www.health.com/ weight-loss/omad-diet

Bendix, A. (2019). 8 signs your intermittent fasting diet has become unsafe or unhealthy. Retrieved from https://www. businessinsider.com/signs-intermittent-fasting-unsafe-unhealthy-2019-7

Berardi, J. (2015). Intermittent Fasting: Whos It For? (And, if Its Not for You, What to Do Instead). Retrieved from https:// www.huffpost.com/entry/intermittent-fasting-whos_b_6236712

Biswas , C. (2020). The One Meal A Day Diet (OMAD Diet) – How It Works, Health Benefits, And Safety. Retrieved from https://www.stylecraze.com/articles/one-meal-a-day-diet-the-ultimate-guide/

Blindow, A. (2019). Fasting: the body's natural stem cell therapy. Retrieved from https://www.intelligent.life/blog/fast-bodys-natural-stem-cell-therapy

Brusie, C. (2017). Is Eating One Meal a Day a Safe and Effective Way to Lose Weight? Retrieved from https://www.healthline.com/health/one-meal-a-day

Carstensen, M. (2018). Intermittent Fasting Helps Reverse Type 2 Diabetes in 3 Men: Study: Everyday Health. Retrieved from https://www.everydayhealth.com/type-2-diabetes/diet/intermittent-fasting-helps-reverse-type-2-diabetes-men-study/

Carter, S., Clifton, P. M., & Keogh, J. B. (2018). Effect of Intermittent vs Continuous Energy Restricted Diet on Glycemic Control in Type 2 Diabetes. Retrieved from https://jamanetwork.com/journals/jamanetworkopen/fullarticle/2688344

Chaix, A., Zarrinpar, A., Miu, P., & Panda, S. (2014). Time-Restricted Feeding Is a Preventative and Therapeutic Intervention against Diverse Nutritional Challenges. Retrieved from https://www.sciencedirect.com/science/article/pii/S1550413114004987?via=ihub

Chander, R. (2018). I Tried Extreme Fasting by Eating Once a Day — Here's What Happened. Retrieved from https://www. healthline.com/health/food-nutrition/one-meal-a-day-diet#1

Cole, W. (2019). OMAD Is The Biggest New Diet Trend For Decreasing Inflammation & Increasing Longevity. Retrieved from https://www.mindbodygreen.com/articles/omad-diet-what-it-is-if-its-safe-and-how-to-do-it

Common Dos and Don'ts of eating One Meal a Day (OMAD) - Times of India. (2019). Retrieved from https://timesofindia. indiatimes.com/life-style/health-fitness/diet/common-dos-and-donts-of-eating-one-meal-a-day-omad/articleshow/ 70805234.cms

Cording, J. (2019). Is the Secret to Losing Weight More About When You Eat Than What? Retrieved from https://www. shape.com/healthy-eating/diet-tips/potential-intermittent-fasting-benefits-not-worth-dieting-risks

de Cabo, R., & Mattson, M. P. (2019). Effects of Intermittent Fasting on Health, Aging, and Disease. Retrieved from https:// www.gwern.net/docs/longevity/2019-decabo.pdf

de Groot, S., Pijl, H., van der Hoeven, J. J. M., & Kroep, J. R. (2019). Effects of short-term fasting on cancer treatment. Retrieved from https://jeccr.biomedcentral.com/articles/10. 1186/s13046-019-1189-9

DeSantis, S. (2019). 30 Minute Vegan Breakfast Burritos. Retrieved from https://www.veggiesdontbite.com/30-minute-vegan-breakfast-burritos-minimalist-baker-everyday-cooking/

Denton, M. (2019). Anti-Aging Benefits of Intermittent Fasting. Retrieved from https://neurohacker.com/anti-aging-benefits-of-intermittent-fasting

Descamps, O., Riondel, J., Ducros, V., & Roussel, A.-M. (2005). Mitochondrial production of reactive oxygen species and incidence of age-associated lymphoma in OF1 mice: effect of alternate-day fasting. Retrieved from https://www.ncbi.nlm.nih.gov/pubmed/16126250

Diet Review: Intermittent Fasting for Weight Loss. (2019). Retrieved from https://www.hsph.harvard.edu/nutritionsource/healthy-weight/diet-reviews/intermittent-fasting/

Duan, W., Guo, Z., Jiang, H., Ware, M., Li, X.-J., & Mattson, M. P. (2003). Dietary restriction normalizes glucose metabolism and BDNF levels, slows disease progression, and increases survival in huntingtin mutant mice. Retrieved from https://www.ncbi.nlm.nih.gov/pmc/articles/PMC151440/

Easy Full English Keto Breakfast: KetoDiet Blog. (2020). Retrieved from https://ketodietapp.com/Blog/lchf/easy-full-english-keto-breakfast

Easy Pork Chops With Asparagus and Hollandaise: KetoDiet Blog. (2020). Retrieved from https://ketodietapp. com/Blog/lchf/easy-pork-chops-with-asparagus-and-hollandaise

Effects of Intermittent Fasting on Health, Aging, and Disease. (2020). Retrieved from https://www.crossfit.com/essentials/effects-of-intermittent-fasting-on-health-aging-and-disease

Eldridge, L. (2019). Can Intermittent Fasting Help Treat or Prevent Cancer? Retrieved from https://www.verywellhealth.com/intermittent-fasting-and-cancer-4772239

Exton, L. (2020). Quick Keto Salmon Power Bowl: KetoDiet Blog. Retrieved from https://ketodietapp.com/Blog/lchf/quick-keto-salmon-power-bowl

Fessenden, M. (2015). Mostly the Old And Ill Ate Breakfast Until the Rise of the Working Man. Retrieved from https://www.smithsonianmag.com/smart-news/mostly-old-and-ill-ate-breakfast-until-rise-working-man-180954041/

Fletcher, J. (2020). One meal a day: Health benefits and risks. Retrieved from https://www.medicalnewstoday.com/articles/320125

Fung, J. (2016). How to Renew Your Body: Fasting and Autophagy. Retrieved from https://www.dietdoctor.com/renew-body-fasting-autophagy

Furmli, S., Elmasry, R., Ramos, M., & Fung, J. (2017). Therapeutic use of intermittent fasting for people with type 2 diabetes as an alternative to insulin. Retrieved from https://casereports. bmj.com/content/2018/bcr-2017-221854.full

Gleeson, J. R. (2019). Intermittent Fasting: Is it Right for You? Retrieved from https://healthblog.uofmhealth.org/wellness-prevention/intermittent-fasting-it-right-for-you

Gleeson, J. R. (2019). Intermittent Fasting: Is it Right for You? Retrieved from https://healthblog.uofmhealth.org/wellness-prevention/intermittent-fasting-it-right-for-you

Goodrick, Charles L., I., K., D., A., M., Freeman, R., J., ... Reynolds. (1983). Differential Effects of Intermittent Feeding and Voluntary Exercise on Body Weight and Lifespan in Adult Rats 1. Retrieved from https://academic.oup.com/geronj/article-abstract/38/1/36/570019

Gunnars, K. (2020). 6 Popular Ways to Do Intermittent Fasting. Retrieved from https://www.healthline.com/nutrition/6-ways-to-do-intermittent-fasting

Gunnars, K. (2017). How Intermittent Fasting Can Help You Lose Weight. Retrieved from https://www.healthline.com/nutrition/intermittent-fasting-and-weight-loss

Gunnars, K. (2016). 10 Evidence-Based Health Benefits of Intermittent Fasting. Retrieved from https://www.healthline.com/nutrition/10-health-benefits-of-intermittent-fasting

Haridy, R. (2019). Review of intermittent fasting research suggests broad health benefits. Retrieved from https://newatlas.

com/health-wellbeing/review-intermittent-fasting-research-health-benefits-johns-hopkins/

Hine, C., Harputlugil , E., Zhang , Y., Ruckenstuhl , C., Cheon Lee , B., Brace , L., ... Mitchell, J. R. (2014). Endogenous Hydrogen Sulfide Production Is Essential for Dietary Restriction Benefits. Retrieved from https://www.cell.com/cell/fulltext/S0092-8674(14)01525-6

How to start OMAD - One Meal a Day. (2018). Retrieved from https://desireepeeples.com/start-omad-one-meal-day/

Intermittent Fasting: 4 Different Types Explained. (2019). Retrieved from https://health.clevelandclinic.org/intermittent-fasting-4-different-types-explained/

Jarreau, P. B. (2018). Eating (Or rather, Fasting) Our Way to Rejuvenated Stem Cells? Retrieved from https://medium.com/lifeomic/eating-or-rather-fasting-our-way-to-rejuvenated-stem-cells-e4302a49e597

Johnson, J. B., Summer, W., Cutler, R. G., Martin, B., Hyun, D.-H., Dixit, V. D., ... Mattson, M. P. (2007). Alternate day calorie restriction improves clinical findings and markers of oxidative stress and inflammation in overweight adults with moderate asthma. Retrieved from https://www.ncbi.nlm.nih.gov/pubmed/17291990/

Johnstone, A. (2015). Fasting for weight loss: an effective strategy or latest dieting trend? Retrieved from https://www.

ncbi.nlm.nih.gov/pubmed/25540982

Jordan , S., Tung , N., Casanova-Acebes , M., Chang , C., Cantoni , C., Zhang , D., ... Merad, M. (2019). Dietary Intake Regulates the Circulating Inflammatory Monocyte Pool. Retrieved from https://www.cell.com/cell/fulltext/S0092-8674(19)30850-5

Kerndt, P. R., Naughton, J. L., Driscoll, C. E., & Loxterkamp, D. A. (1982). Fasting: the history, pathophysiology and complications. Retrieved from https://www.ncbi.nlm.nih.gov/pubmed/6758355

Landsverk, G. (2019). Intermittent fasting may help slow aging and diseases like cancer and diabetes - even if you don't lose weight. Retrieved from https://www.insider.com/intermittent-fasting-slows-aging-cancer-diabetes-heart-disease-study-2019-12

Lee, C., Raffaghello, L., Brandhorst, S., Safdie, F. M., Bianchi, G., Martin-Montalvo, A., ... Longo, V. D. (2012). Fasting cycles retard growth of tumors and sensitize a range of cancer cell types to chemotherapy. Retrieved from https://www.ncbi.nlm.nih.gov/pubmed/22323820

Lee, J., Duan, W., Long, J. M., Ingram, D. K., & Mattson, M. P. (2000). Dietary restriction increases the number of newly generated neural cells, and induces BDNF expression, in the dentate gyrus of rats. Retrieved from https://www.ncbi.nlm.nih.gov/pubmed/11220789

Leech, J. (2019). 5 Stats That Show Why Intermittent Fasting is Powerful for Weight Loss. Retrieved from https://www. dietvsdisease.org/intermittent-fasting-is-powerful-for-weight-loss/

Leonard, J. (2020). 7 formas de hacer ayuno intermitente: Los mejores métodos. Retrieved from https://www. medicalnewstoday.com/articles/322293

Levy, J. (2018). Benefits of Autophagy, Plus How to Induce It. Retrieved from https://draxe.com/health/benefits-of-autophagy/

Li, L., Wang, Z., & Zuo, Z. (2013). Chronic intermittent fasting improves cognitive functions and brain structures in mice. Retrieved from https://www.ncbi.nlm.nih.gov/pmc/articles/PMC3670843/

Lindberg, S. (2018). Autophagy: What You Need to Know. Retrieved from https://www.healthline.com/health/autophagy

London, J. (2019, May 28). The Trendy OMAD Diet Has a Ton of Potentially Scary Side Effects. Retrieved from https://www. goodhousekeeping.com/health/diet-nutrition/a27506052/omad-diet/

Low-Carb Steak Taco Bowl: KetoDiet Blog. (2020). Retrieved from https://ketodietapp.com/Blog/lchf/low-carb-steak-taco-bowl

Magyar, O. (2017). Intermittent Fasting For Better Brain Health? Retrieved from https://neurotrition.ca/blog/intermittent-fasting-better-brain-health

Marosi, K., Moehl , K., Navas-Enamorado, I., Mitchell, S. J., Zhang, Y., Lehrmann , E., ... Mattson, M. P. (2018). Metabolic and molecular framework for the enhancement of endurance by intermittent food deprivation. Retrieved from https://www.fasebj.org/doi/10.1096/fj.201701378RR

Mattson, M. P., Moehl, K., Ghena, N., Schmaedick, M., & Cheng, A. (2018). Intermittent metabolic switching, neuroplasticity and brain health. Retrieved from https://www.ncbi.nlm.nih.gov/pubmed/29321682

Mattson, M. P. (2005). Energy intake, meal frequency, and health: a neurobiological perspective. Retrieved from https://www.ncbi.nlm.nih.gov/pubmed/16011467

McLeod, C. (2019). Intermittent fasting is trendy but dietitians warn against it. Retrieved from https://www.bodyandsoul.com.au/nutrition/nutrition-tips/the-6-people-who-shouldnt-try-intermittent-fasting-according-to-a-dietitian/news-story/ca97f74fc904811f4b78281824dea72c

Migala, J. (2020). 7 Types of Intermittent Fasting: Which Is Best for You?: Everyday Health. Retrieved from https://www.everydayhealth.com/diet-nutrition/diet/types-intermittent-fasting-which-best-you/

Mihaylova, M. M., Cheng, C.-W., Cao, A. Q., Tripathi, S., Mana, M. D., Bauer-Rowe, K. E., ... Yilmaz, Ö. H. (2018). Fasting Activates Fatty Acid Oxidation to Enhance Intestinal Stem Cell Function during Homeostasis and Aging. Retrieved from https://www.sciencedirect.com/science/article/pii/S1934590918301632

Moller, N., Vendelbo, M. H., Kampmann, U., Christensen, B., Madsen, M., Norrelund, H., & Jorgensen, J. O. (2009). Growth hormone and protein metabolism. Retrieved from https://www.ncbi.nlm.nih.gov/pubmed/19773097

Moro, T., Tinsley, G., Bianco, A., Marcolin, G., Pacelli, Q. F., Battaglia, G., ... Paoli, A. (2016). Effects of eight weeks of time-restricted feeding (16/8) on basal metabolism, maximal strength, body composition, inflammation, and cardiovascular risk factors in resistance-trained males. Retrieved from https://translational-medicine.biomedcentral.com/articles/10.1186/s12967-016-1044-0

Nørrelund, H., Nair, K. S., Jørgensen, J. O., Christiansen, J. S., & Møller, N. (2001). The protein-retaining effects of growth hormone during fasting involve inhibition of muscle-protein breakdown. Retrieved from https://www.ncbi.nlm.nih.gov/pubmed/11147801

O'Flanagan, C. H., Smith, L. A., McDonell, S. B., & Hursting, S. D. (2017). When less may be more: calorie restriction and response to cancer therapy. Retrieved from https://www.ncbi.nlm.nih.gov/pubmed/28539118

OMAD DIET: THE ULTIMATE GUIDE. (2019). Retrieved from https://omadmealplan.com/

Oppenheim, S. (2019). Is Intermittent Fasting Really The Healthiest Way To Eat? Not For Everyone. Retrieved from https://www.forbes.com/sites/serenaoppenheim/2019/01/24/is-intermittent-fasting-really-the-healthiest-way-to-eat-not-for-everyone/#276fd2d13606

Paddock, C. (2018). How fasting boosts exercise's effects on endurance. Retrieved from https://www.medicalnewstoday.com/articles/321056

Park, M. (2010). Nearing 50, Renaissance jock Herschel Walker breaks fitness rules. Retrieved from http://edition.cnn.com/2010/HEALTH/10/11/herschel.fitness.martial.arts/index.html

Pattillo, A. (2019). The Truth Behind What Intermittent Fasting Does to Your Body. Retrieved from https://www.inverse.com/article/57625-what-intermittent-fasting-actually-does-to-your-body

Pawlowski, A. (2019). What is the OMAD diet? Learn how the one-meal-a-day plan works. Retrieved from https://www.today.com/health/what-omad-diet-learn-how-one-meal-day-diet-works-t146204

Permanente, K. (n.d.). How our bodies turn food into energy. Retrieved from https://wa.kaiserpermanente.org/healthAndWellness?item=/common/healthAndWellness/conditions/diabetes/foodProcess.html

Pleimling, A. (2017). Trendy or troublesome? Get the facts on intermittent fasting. Retrieved from https://www.allinahealth.org/healthysetgo/nourish/trendy-or-troublesome-the-facts-on-intermittent-fasting

Phillips, M. C. L. (2019). Fasting as a Therapy in Neurological Disease. Retrieved from https://www.ncbi.nlm.nih.gov/pmc/articles/PMC6836141/

Presto, G. (2017). Is Intermittent Fasting Right For You? Retrieved from https://www.bornfitness.com/intermittent-fasting/

Research on intermittent fasting shows health benefits. (2020, February 27). Retrieved from https://www.nia.nih.gov/news/research-intermittent-fasting-shows-health-benefits

Researchers discover that fasting reduces inflammation and improves chronic inflammatory diseases. (2019). Retrieved from https://medicalxpress.com/news/2019-08-fasting-inflammation-chronic-inflammatory-diseases.html

Ries, J. (2020). This Is Your Body On Intermittent Fasting. Retrieved from https://www.huffpost.com/entry/body-intermittent-fasting_l_5e0a3220c5b6b5a713b22dcb?

guccounter=1&guce_referrer=

aHR0cHM6Ly93d3cuZ29vZ2xlLmNvbS8&guce_referrer_sig=

AQAAAC-

HM3NWPXeuZI89BsKO_6IpI8l9andTLuWwBQJfgG-

AsuIWgujK_56SnSe6nwtztpxQJ50POffVrpAasbAvte9Zq5Z31

m4DPBrmQfjl-gS1ahKuyRQNZApPT-

6VAiMjRY5SqN1g6Vcfx_jg2BiwVYsMz8SklicgTXv6h1SZI-GS

Rinzler, C. A., & DeVault, K. (n.d.). The Human Digestion
Process (or, What Happens after You Eat Food). Retrieved from
https://www.dummies.com/education/science/biology/the-
human-digestion-process-or-what-happens-after-you-eat-
food/

Rose, E. (2020). OMAD: What is One Meal a Day Fasting, and
Should You Try It? Retrieved from https://www.bulletproof.
com/diet/intermittent-fasting/omad-one-meal-a-day-diet/

Rumi Quote: "Fasting is the first principle of medicine; fast and
see the strength of the spirit reveal itself.". (n.d.). Retrieved
from https://quotefancy.com/quote/904488/Rumi-Fasting-is-
the-first-principle-of-medicine-fast-and-see-the-strength-of-
the-spirit

Save, K. (2019). What really happens to your body during intermittent fasting. Retrieved from https://www.bodyandsoul.com.
au/diet/diets/what-really-happens-to-your-body-during-
intermittent-fasting/news-
story/92cdbf27507d9fa3afe30eaab3172b5e

Scher, B. (2020). What You Need to Know About OMAD. Retrieved from https://www.dietdoctor.com/intermittent-fasting/omad

Schmidt, M. (2020). What Science Says About the Weight-Loss Potential of 'OMAD' Fasting - The One-Meal-a-Day Diet. Retrieved from https://www.discovermagazine.com/health/what-science-says-about-the-weight-loss-potential-of-omad-fasting-the-one

Seimon, R. V., Roekenes, J. A., Zibellini, J., Zhu, B., Gibson, A. A., Hills, A. P., ... Sainsbury, A. (2015). Do intermittent diets provide physiological benefits over continuous diets for weight loss? A systematic review of clinical trials. Retrieved from https://www.sciencedirect.com/science/article/abs/pii/S0303720715300800?via=ihub

Sigurdsson, A. F. (2020). Intermittent Fasting and Health – The Scientific Evidence. Retrieved from https://www.docsopinion.com/intermittent-fasting

Sisson, M. (2020). 7 Tips and Considerations for Eating One Meal a Day. Retrieved from https://www.marksdailyapple.com/7-tips-and-considerations-for-eating-one-meal-a-day/

Sogawa, H., & Kubo, C. (2000). Influence of short-term repeated fasting on the longevity of female (NZB×NZW)F1 mice. Retrieved from https://www.sciencedirect.com/science/article/abs/pii/S0047637400001093

Southard, L. (2020). What is OMAD diet: Why eating one meal a day isn't recommended by experts. Retrieved from https://www.insider.com/what-is-omad-diet

Stieg, C. (2019). Is The OMAD Diet The New Intermittent Fasting? Retrieved from https://www.refinery29.com/en-us/eating-one-meal-a-day-diet-trend

Stote, K. S., Baer, D. J., Spears, K., Paul, D. R., Harris, G. K., Rumpler, W. V., … Mattson, M. P. (2007). A controlled trial of reduced meal frequency without caloric restriction in healthy, normal-weight, middle-aged adults. Retrieved from https://www.ncbi.nlm.nih.gov/pmc/articles/PMC2645638/

Sweet Potato Taco Bowl. (2019). Retrieved from https://www.mykitchenlove.com/sweet-potato-taco-bowl/

Tello, M. (2020). Intermittent fasting: Surprising update. Retrieved from https://www.health.harvard.edu/blog/intermittent-fasting-surprising-update-2018062914156

Templeman, I., Gonzalez, J. T., Thompson, D., & Betts, J. A. (2020). The role of intermittent fasting and meal timing in weight management and metabolic health. Retrieved from https://www.ncbi.nlm.nih.gov/pubmed/31023390

Templeton, L. (2019). Intermittent fasting can help ease metabolic syndrome. Retrieved from https://www.medicalnewstoday.com/articles/327247

The Dangers of Intermittent Fasting. (2019). Retrieved from https://centerfordiscovery.com/blog/the-dangers-of-intermittent-fasting/

The OMAD Diet: Is Having One Meal A Day Effective? (2020). Retrieved from https://betterme.world/articles/omad-diet/

The Warrior Diet: Review and Beginner's Guide. (2018). Retrieved from https://www.healthline.com/nutrition/warrior-diet-guide

Tinsley, G. M., & La Bounty, P. M. (2015). Effects of intermittent fasting on body composition and clinical health markers in humans. Retrieved from https://academic.oup.com/nutritionreviews/article/73/10/661/1849182

Top 10 Tips for OMAD - Tips for One Meal a Day Diet. (2019). Retrieved from http://siimland.com/top-10-tips-for-omad-tips-for-one-meal-a-day-diet/

Varady, K. A., & Hellerstein, M. K. (2007). Alternate-day fasting and chronic disease prevention: a review of human and animal trials. Retrieved from https://www.ncbi.nlm.nih.gov/pubmed/17616757?dopt=Abstract

Varady, K. A., Bhutani, S., Church, E. C., & Klempel, M. C. (2009). Short-term modified alternate-day fasting: a novel dietary strategy for weight loss and cardioprotection in obese adults. Retrieved from https://www.ncbi.nlm.nih.gov/pubmed/19793855

Varady, K. A. (2011). Intermittent versus daily calorie restriction: which diet regimen is more effective for weight loss? Retrieved from https://www.ncbi.nlm.nih.gov/pubmed/21410865

Weindruch, R., & Sohal, R. S. (1997). Seminars in medicine of the Beth Israel Deaconess Medical Center. Caloric intake and aging. Retrieved from https://www.ncbi.nlm.nih.gov/pmc/articles/PMC2851235/

West, H. (2016). Does Intermittent Fasting Boost Your Metabolism? Retrieved from https://www.healthline.com/nutrition/intermittent-fasting-metabolism

What happens to the food we eat? - (Food and Body Function). (n.d.). Retrieved from http://apjcn.nhri.org.tw/server/info/books-phds/books/foodfacts/html/maintext/main3a.html

Wilkinson, M. J., Manoogian, E. N. C., Zadourian, A., Navlakha, S., Lo, H., Fakhouri, S., ... Taub, P. R. (2019). Ten-Hour Time-Restricted Eating Reduces Weight, Blood Pressure, and Atherogenic Lipids in Patients with Metabolic Syndrome. Retrieved from https://www.cell.com/cell-metabolism/fulltext/S1550-4131(19)30611-4

Zahid, U. (2019). (Ultimate Guide) All You Need to Know About OMAD Diet. Retrieved from https://ashrafchaudhryblog.com/omad-diet/

Zarrinpar, A., Chaix, A., Yooseph, S., & Panda, S. (2014). Diet and feeding pattern affect the diurnal dynamics of the gut microbiome. Retrieved from https://www.ncbi.nlm.nih.gov/pubmed/25470548

Zhang, J., Zhan, Z., Li, X., Xing, A., Jiang, C., Chen, Y., ... An, L. (2017). Intermittent Fasting Protects against Alzheimer's Disease Possible through Restoring Aquaporin-4 Polarity. Retrieved from https://www.ncbi.nlm.nih.gov/pmc/articles/PMC5712566/

REFERENCES

Alirezaei, M., Kemball, C. C., Flynn, C. T., Wood, M. R., Whitton, J. L., & Kiosses, W. B. (2010, August). Short-term fasting induces profound neuronal autophagy. *Autophagy*, 6(6), 702-710. https://doi.org/10.4161/auto.6.6.12376

Anson, R. M., Guo, Z., de Cabo, R., Iyun, T., Rios, M., Hagepanos, A., ... Mattson, M. P. (2003, May 13). Intermittent fasting dissociates beneficial effects of dietary restriction on glucose metabolism and neuronal resistance to injury from calorie intake. *Proceedings of the National Academy of Sciences of the United States of America*, 100(10), 6216-6220. https://doi.org/10.1073/pnas.1035720100

Beleslin, B., Cirić, J., Zarković, M., Vujović, S., Trbojević, B., & Drezgić, M. (2007). The effects of three-week fasting diet on blood pressure, lipid profile and glucoregulation in extremely obese patients. *Srpski Arhiv Za Celokupno Lekarstvo, 135*(7-8), 440-446. https://doi.org/10.2298/sarh0708440b.

Brandhorst, S., Choi, I. Y., Wei, M., Cheng, C. W., Sedrakyan, S., Navarrete, G., ... Longo, V. D. (2015, July 7). A periodic diet that mimics fasting promotes multi-system regeneration, enhanced cognitive performance, and healthspan. *Cell Metabolism, 22*(1), 86-99. https://doi.org/10.1016/j.cmet.2015.05.012

Gunnars, K. (2019, July 24). *Insulin and insulin resistance - The ultimate guide.* Healthline. https://www.healthline.com/nutrition/insulin-and-insulin-resistance

Hunter, P. (2012, November 6). The inflammation theory of disease. The growing realization that chronic inflammation is crucial in many diseases opens new avenues for treatment. *EMBO Reports, 13*(11), 968-970. https://doi.org/10.1038/embor.2012.142

Kmiec, Z., Pokrywka, L., Kotlarz, G., Kubasik, J., Szutowicz, A., & Mysliwski, A. (2005). Effects of fasting and refeeding on serum leptin, adiponectin and free fatty acid concentrations in young and old male rats. *Gerontology, 51*(6), 357-362. https://doi.org/10.1159/000088698

Lee, J., Duan, W., Long, J. M., Ingram, D. K., & Mattson, M. P. (2000, October). Dietary restriction increases the number of newly generated neural cells, and induces BDNF expression, in the dentate gyrus of rats. *Journal of Molecular*

Neuroscience, 15(2), 99-108. https://doi.org/10.1385/
JMN:15:2:99

Levine, B., & Kroemer, G. (2008, January 11). Autophagy in the pathogenesis of disease. *Cell, 132*(1), 27-72. https://doi.org/10.1016/j.cell.2007.12.018

Li, L., Wang, Z., & Zuo, Z. (2013, June 3). Chronic intermittent fasting improves cognitive functions and brain structures in mice. *PloS One, 8*(6), e66069. https://doi.org/10.1371/journal.pone.0066069.

The Nobel Prize in physiology or medicine 2016. (2016). NobelPrize.Org. https://www.nobelprize.org/prizes/medicine/2016/press-release/

Purvis, J. (2009, July 6). Suffragette hunger strikes, 100 years on. *The Guardian.* https://www.theguardian.com/commentisfree/libertycentral/2009/jul/06/suffragette-hunger-strike-protest

Raman, R. (2019, December 18). *Water fasting.* Healthline. https://www.healthline.com/nutrition/water-fasting

Rose, K. (n.d.). *The mental health benefits of fasting.* Amchara. https://www.amchara.com/diet-fasting/the-mental-health-benefits-of-fasting

Salgin, B., (2012, April 1). The effect of prolonged fasting on levels of growth hormone-binding protein and free growth hormone. *Growth Hormone & IGF Research: Official Journal of the Growth Hormone Research Society and the*

International IGF Research Society, 22(2), 76-81. https://doi.org/10.1016/j.ghir.2012.02.003

Short history of fasting. (2017, June 5). Target Health. https://www.targethealth.com/post/short-history-of-fasting

Staff, S. X. (2019, August 22). *Researchers discover that fasting reduces inflammation and improves chronic inflammatory diseases.* Medical Xpress. https://medicalxpress.com/news/2019-08-fasting-inflammation-chronic-inflammatory-diseases.html

Tinsley, G. M., & La Bounty, P. M. (2015, October). Effects of intermittent fasting on body composition and clinical health markers in humans. *Nutrition Reviews, 73*(10), 661-674. https://doi.org/10.1093/nutrit/nuv041

Water fasting (benefits & how to break the fast). (2020, February 4). The LifeCo. https://www.thelifeco.com/en/blog/common-questions-about-water-fasting-benefits-how-to-break-the-fast/

Watson, S. (2020, February 27). *Diabetes: Symptoms, causes, treatment, prevention, and more.* Healthline. https://www.healthline.com/health/diabetes

Wellman, J., (2015). *24 William Secker Quotes.* Christian Quotes. https://www.christianquotes.info/quotes-by-author/william-secker-quotes/

Zauner, C., Schneeweiss, B., Kranz, A., Madl, C., Ratheiser, K., Kramer, L., ... Lenz, K. (2000, June). Resting energy expenditure in short-term starvation is increased as a result of an increase in serum norepinephrine. *The American Journal of Clinical Nutrition, 71*(6), 1511-1515. https://doi.org/10.1093/ajcn/71.6.1511

IMAGE REFERENCE LIST

All images have been sourced from https://pixabay.com

Figure 1: Child Praying. From Pixabay, by Chidioc, 2017. https://pixabay.com/photos/kid-praying-muslim-islam-faith-1077793/

Figure 2: Mineral Water. From Pixabay, by Congerdesign, 2019. https://pixabay.com/photos/bottle-mineral-water-bottle-of-water-2032980/

Figure 3: Pregnancy. From Pixabay, by Free-Photos, 2019. pixabay.com/photos/pregnant-mother-body-pregnant-woman-1245703/

Figure 4: Heart Health. From Pixabay, by InspiredImages, 2017. https://pixabay.com/photos/heart-care-medical-care-heart-1040250/

Figure 5: Yoga. From Pixabay, by StockSnap, 2020. pixabay.com/photos/people-woman-yoga-meditation-2573216/

Figure 6: Orange Juice. From Pixabay, by Stevepb, 2020. https://pixabay.com/photos/fresh-orange-juice-squeezed-1614822/

Figure 7: Scrambled Eggs. From Pixabay, by Maki_Orel, 2017. https://pixabay.com/photos/breakfast-scrambled-eggs-bun-chive-876432/

Figure 8: Muscle Mass. From Pixabay, by Ryan McGuire, 2019. https://pixabay.com/photos/man-muscle-fitness-workout-641691/

Figure 9: Abdominal Pain. From Pixabay, by Derneuemann, 2020.   https://pixabay.com/photos/abdominal-pain-pain-appendicitis-2821941/

Figure 10: Brushing teeth. From Pixabay, by Stevepb, 2020. https://pixabay.com/photos/toothbrush-toothpaste-dental-care-571741/

CPSIA information can be obtained
at www.ICGtesting.com
Printed in the USA
LVHW051357130721
692565LV00006B/520